New Knowledge about Pulmonary Thromoboembolism

Edited by Jelena Stojšić

Published in London, United Kingdom

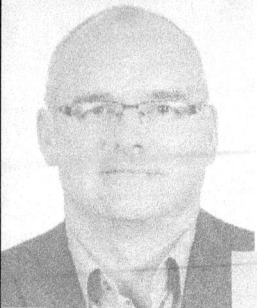
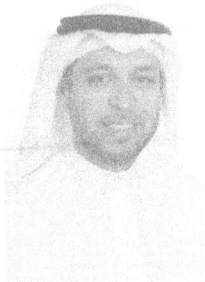
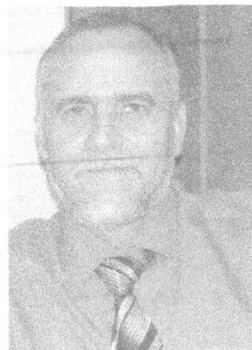
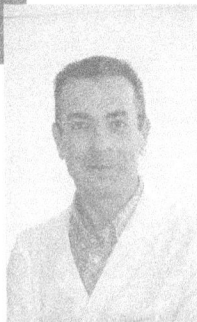
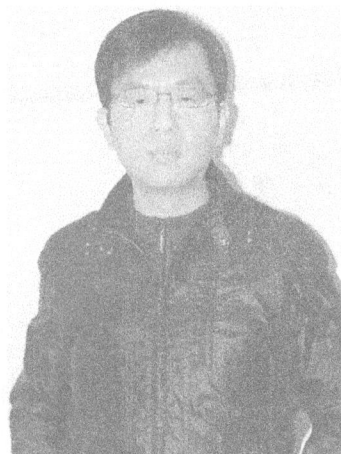
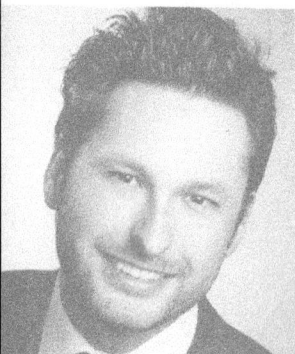
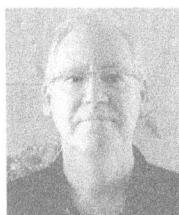

IntechOpen

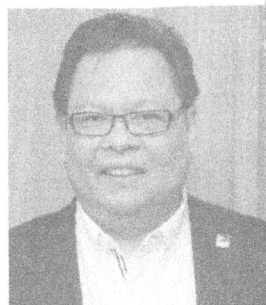
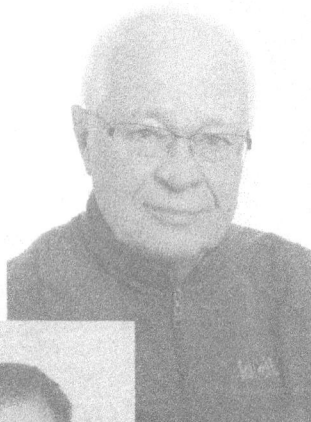
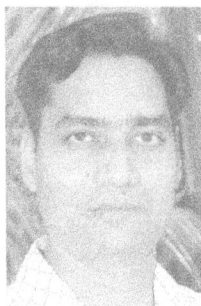
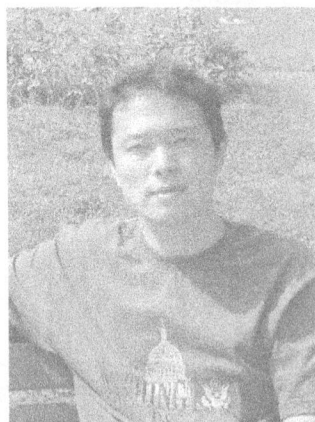
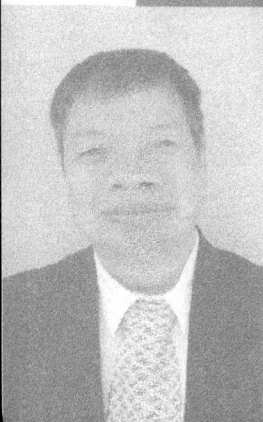
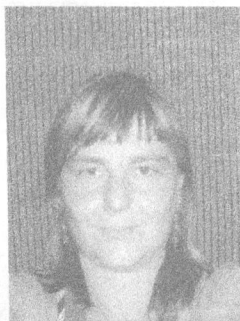

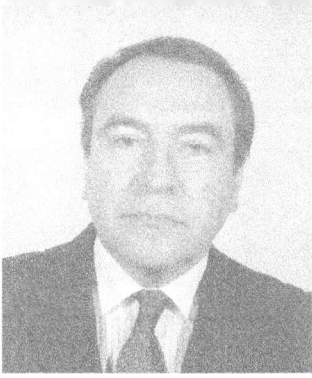

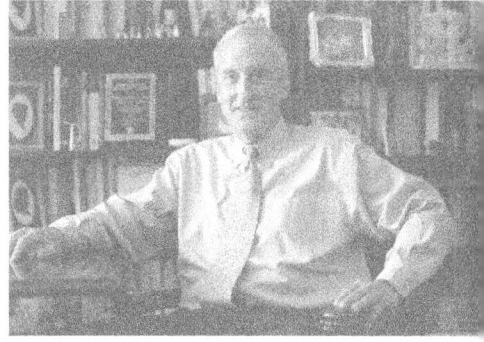

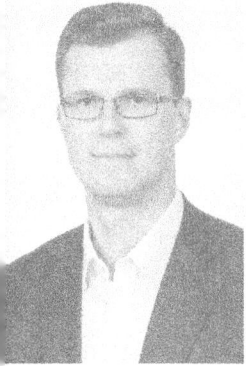

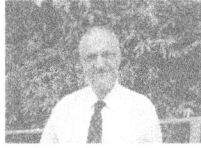

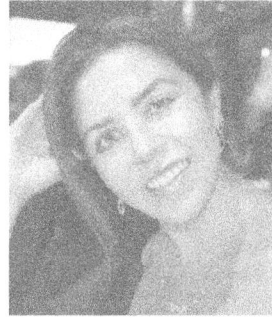

Supporting open minds since 2005

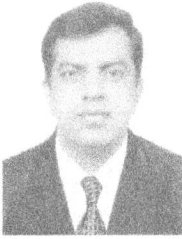

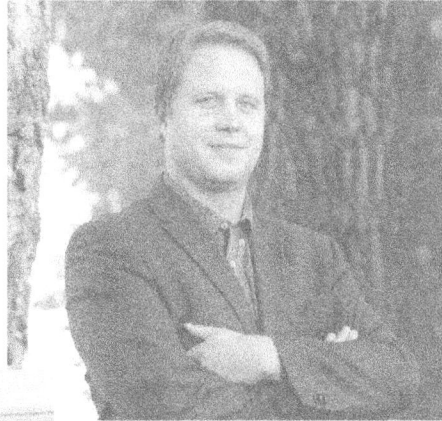

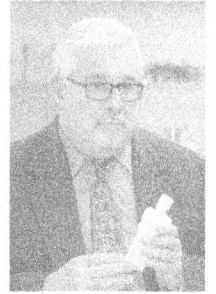

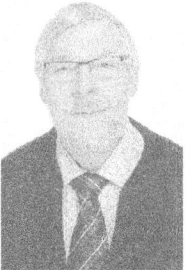

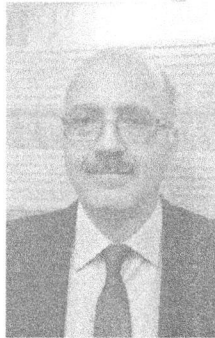

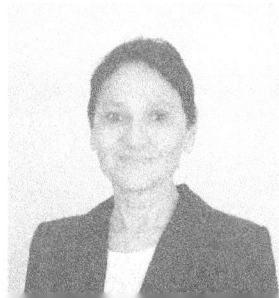

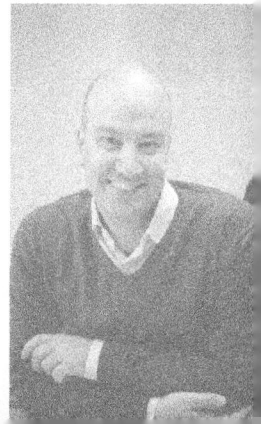

New Knowledge about Pulmonary Thromoboembolism
http://dx.doi.org/10.5772/intechopen.94698
Edited by Jelena Stojšić

Contributors
Sachin M. Patil, Nissar Shaikh, Narges Quyyum, Muhammad Zubair, Muhsen Shaheen, Sumayya Aboobacker, Jazib Hassan, Zubair Shahid, Shajahan Idayathulla, Ashish Kumar, Ibrahim Rasheed, Arshad Chanda, Shoaib Nawaz, M.M. Nainthramveetil, Ladan Panahi, George Udeani, Michael Horseman, Jaye Weston, Nephy Samuel, Merlyn Joseph, Andrea Mora, Daniela Bazan, Pooja Patel, Navdeep Singh Sidhu, Sumandeep Kaur, Cynthia Sadera, Sharon Halliburton

Notice
Statements and opinions expressed in the chapters are these of the individual contributors and not necessarily those of the editors or publisher. No responsibility is accepted for the accuracy of information contained in the published chapters. The publisher assumes no responsibility for any damage or injury to persons or property arising out of the use of any materials, instructions, methods or ideas contained in the book.

First published in London, United Kingdom, 2022 by IntechOpen
IntechOpen is the global imprint of INTECHOPEN LIMITED, registered in England and Wales, registration number: 11086078, 5 Princes Gate Court, London, SW7 2QJ, United Kingdom
Printed in Croatia

British Library Cataloguing-in-Publication Data
A catalogue record for this book is available from the British Library

Additional hard and PDF copies can be obtained from orders@intechopen.com

New Knowledge about Pulmonary Thromoboembolism
Edited by Jelena Stojšić
p. cm.
Print ISBN 978-1-83969-966-5
Online ISBN 978-1-83969-967-2
eBook (PDF) ISBN 978-1-83969-968-9

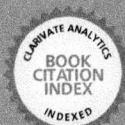

Meet the editor

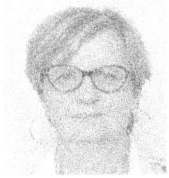

Jelena Stojšić is a senior scientific researcher and has been a thoracic pathologist for the last 28 years. Her major interest is in the field of lung pathology, particularly in lung cancer, pleural tumors, and interstitial and vascular lung diseases. The aim of her Ph.D. thesis was to recognize the link between molecular pathways in lung cancer and transport pumps involved in the reflux of chemotherapeutics from malignant cells. In daily practice, Dr. Stojšić focuses on the diagnosis of pathological lung cancer based on morphology and immunoprofile for personalized patient therapy. She is also a book author and editor.

Contents

Preface

Pulmonary thromboembolism has appeared as a frequent complication in COVID-19 infection. As such, this book discusses the diagnosis of pulmonary thromboembolism in patients with and without COVID-19. Chapters address such topics as clinical symptoms of the disorder, biochemical and radiological findings in patients with pulmonary thromboembolism, and the modern approach to therapy.

The book is a useful resource for the general population of doctors, particularly internists, pulmonologists, and infectious disease specialists.

Jelena Stojšić, MD Ph.D.
University Clinical Centre of Serbia,
Belgrade, Serbia

Chapter 1

Introductory Chapter: Pulmonary Embolism

Cynthia Sadera, Sharon Halliburton, Ladan Panahi and George Udeani

1. Introduction

Pulmonary embolism (PE) is typically caused by emboli, originating from venous thrombi traveling to and occluding the lung's arteries. These emboli characteristically arise in the leg, referred to as deep vein thrombosis (DVT), which may detach and travel to the pulmonary arteries, halting blood flow, and resulting in tissue ischemia. While there are a variety of etiologies, associated with pulmonary embolism, the most prevalent is DVT. Patients with specific disease states, including blood coagulation disorders, cancer, stroke, paralysis, coronary artery disease, and hypertension, have an increased risk of developing a pulmonary embolism. Surgical procedures and skeletal fractures also threaten the occurrence of coagulation, where the risk of pulmonary embolism tends to increase weeks after either event. Other risk factors include prolonged inactivity, obesity, cigarette use, recent endothelial injury, old age, and hypercoagulable states (cancer). Patients who are pregnant or within 6 weeks of giving birth also carry an increased risk of pulmonary infarction. Certain medications such as oral contraceptives, hormone replacement therapy, and chemotherapeutic agents can also correlate with higher incidences of pulmonary embolism [1]. Virchow triad (stasis, vascular wall injury, and hypercoagulable state) may be employed in the assessment of the risk of thrombi formation [2]. Pulmonary embolism is one of the most dangerous categories of venous thromboembolism, with high fatality rates if undiagnosed or untreated [3]. Furthermore, the post-PE syndrome may occur in individuals who survive PE. This is characterized by chronic thrombotic remains in the pulmonary arteries, tenacious right ventricular dysfunction, decreased quality of life, or chronic functional limitations [4]. Right ventricular dysfunction associated with acute PE can lead to complications such as arrhythmia, hemodynamic collapse, and shock [5].

Acute PE is a major global health concern. Approximately 10 million DVT cases are diagnosed globally annually, with one million cases occurring in the United States and approximately 700,000 in France, Italy, Germany, Spain, Sweden, and the United Kingdom combined annually [6–8]. In the United States, an estimated 100,000 to 200,000 individuals die annually from pulmonary embolism [9]. The incidence of acute PE in China tripled from 3.9 per 100,000 in 2000–2001 to 11.7 per 100,000 in 2010–2011 and is projected to increase, given the expected increase in China's population [10, 11].

Despite its devastating mortality, pulmonary embolism can be prevented, particularly by implementing certain safeguard measures. Such safeguards include lower extremities mobility, particularly during periods of prolonged inactivity, routine exercise, a healthy diet, decreased alcohol, nicotine, and caffeine intake, and early post-surgical ambulation after a recent surgery or medical illness to reduce risks. Prevention of deep vein thrombosis further reduces the risk of pulmonary embolism. Employing compression stockings, sequential compression devices, lifestyle modification to include exercise, and therapeutic agents as prophylactic measures have long-term implications in reducing fatal pulmonary embolism [12]. Pulmonary embolism response teams (PERTs), similar to Code Blue teams employed during emergency cardiopulmonary arrests in hospitals, are emerging globally to mitigate this international PE crisis [13].

Clinical presentation of pulmonary embolism frequently overlaps with other disease states; thus, it is not unusual for pulmonary embolism to be misdiagnosed. Symptoms such as shortness of breath, chest pain, coughing with or without bloody sputum, cardiac arrhythmias, anxiety, cyanosis, lightheadedness, tachypnea, sweating, or tachycardia are symptoms of a pulmonary embolism and a variety of other cardiopulmonary conditions [14]. Other signs such as edema, erythema, pain, or tenderness of the leg may indicate DVT, with a direct risk of pulmonary embolism. Therefore, it is imperative that clinicians pay close attention to the latter in making an accurate diagnosis and thus employing appropriate therapeutic interventions that will yield positive outcomes in these patient populations. The medical history, physical exam, and certain test results are employed for the differential diagnosis of pulmonary embolism from other conditions. Accurate history and physical examination, pertinent lab values such as D-Dimer, employment of leg ultrasound, computed tomography (CT) scan, lung ventilation-perfusion scan, blood tests, echocardiography, chest X-ray, or chest MRI are all avenues employed in the timely and accurate diagnosis, and thus intervention in pulmonary embolism to reduce mortality and improve patient outcomes [15].

Once the diagnosis of a pulmonary embolism is confirmed, it is critical to initiate treatment immediately. Such treatment typically occurs in emergency medicine, or inpatient environments, with the emergent goal of halting the blood clot transit progression and preventing new clot development. A myriad of anticoagulation therapies is currently available to manage pulmonary embolism, ranging from parenteral to oral treatments. Anticoagulation therapy inhibits certain aspects of the clotting cascade to prevent the growth of the clot infarction and avoid additional thrombogenesis. Common anticoagulants employed include heparin, warfarin, and direct-acting oral anticoagulants. It is critical to monitor for signs and symptoms of bleeding, food, and drug interactions, as well as efficacy associated with these treatment modalities, for optimal outcomes. Adverse events to these agents may occur; these include bright red or coffee grounds emesis, black tarry stool, and abdominal pain without attributable cause are all signs of gastrointestinal bleeding. Additionally, patients on such therapies may experience severe headaches, sudden vision changes, sudden loss of movement or feeling in any extremities, memory loss, or disorientation, which are all signs of intracranial bleeding [16].

Other forms of therapy include fibrinolytics, catheter-directed therapies, and surgical embolectomy [17]. Fibrinolytic therapy is indicated in a select group of hemodynamically unstable patients. Surgical therapy in these patients is employed as a last resort. These procedures include inferior vena cava (IVC) filter placement, pulmonary embolectomy, and percutaneous thrombectomy. IVC filter insertion is indicated in patients with medical contraindications to anticoagulation, anticoagulant-induced hypercoagulation, or patients with excessive bleeding risks [18].

Pulmonary embolism is a preventable manifestation of venous thromboembolism which may be misdiagnosed, due to its non-specific symptoms. Pulmonary embolism prevention via lifestyle modification, increased physical exercise, and early employment of prophylactic therapy in at-risk populations are the best approaches. Rapid detection, diagnosis, and early employment of therapeutic or surgical interventions are vital to improving outcomes and decreasing morbidity and mortality.

Author details

Cynthia Sadera[1,2], Sharon Halliburton[1,2], Ladan Panahi[1,2] and George Udeani[1,2]*

1 Department of Pharmacy Practice, Texas A&M Rangel College of Pharmacy, Kingsville, TX, United States

2 Department of Pharmacy Practice, Texas A&M Rangel College of Pharmacy, College Station, TX, United States

*Address all correspondence to: udeani@tamu.edu

IntechOpen

References

[1] Mammen EF. Pathogenesis of venous thrombosis. Chest. 1992;**102**(6): 640S-644S

[2] Watson T, Shantsila E, Lip GY. Mechanisms of thrombogenesis in atrial fibrillation: Virchow's triad revisited. The Lancet. 2009;**373**(9658):155-166

[3] Anderson FA, Wheeler HB, Goldberg RJ, et al. A population-based perspective of the hospital incidence and case-fatality rates of deep vein thrombosis and pulmonary embolism: The Worcester DVT study. Archives of Internal Medicine. 1991;**151**(5): 933-938

[4] Klok F, Van der Hulle T, Den Exter P, Lankeit M, Huisman M, Konstantinides S. The post-PE syndrome: A new concept for chronic complications of pulmonary embolism. Blood Reviews. 2014;**28**(6):221-226

[5] Agnelli G, Becattini C. Acute pulmonary embolism. New England Journal of Medicine. 2010;**363**(3): 266-274

[6] Haider A, Goldberg J. National trends in pulmonary embolism management and outcomes: Shifting paradigms. Journal of the American College of Cardiology. 2019;**73**(9S1): 1901-1901

[7] Horlander KT, Mannino DM, Leeper KV. Pulmonary embolism mortality in the United States, 1979-1998: An analysis using multiple-cause mortality data. Archives of Internal Medicine. 2003;**163**(14):1711-1717

[8] Jha AK, Larizgoitia I, Audera-Lopez C, Prasopa-Plaizier N, Waters H, Bates DW. The global burden of unsafe medical care: Analytic modelling of observational studies. BMJ Quality & Safety. 2013;**22**(10):809-815

[9] Park B, Messina L, Dargon P, Huang W, Ciocca R, Anderson FA. Recent trends in clinical outcomes and resource utilization for pulmonary embolism in the United States: Findings from the nationwide inpatient sample. Chest. 2009;**136**(4):983-990

[10] Yang Y, Liang L, Zhai Z, et al. Pulmonary embolism incidence and fatality trends in Chinese hospitals from 1997 to 2008: A multicenter registration study. PLoS One. 2011;**6**(11):e26861

[11] Law Y, Chan YC, Cheng SW. Epidemiological updates of venous thromboembolism in a Chinese population. Asian Journal of Surgery. 2018;**41**(2):176-182

[12] Young T, Sriram KB. Vena caval filters for the prevention of pulmonary embolism. Cochrane Database of Systematic Reviews. 2020;**10**(10): CD006212. Pages 1-59. Published October 8, 2020. DOI: 10.1002/14651858. CD006212.pub5

[13] Kabrhel C, Rosovsky R, Channick R, et al. A multidisciplinary pulmonary embolism response team: Initial 30-month experience with a novel approach to delivery of care to patients with submassive and massive pulmonary embolism. Chest. 2016;**150**(2):384-393

[14] Kwok CS, Wong CW, Lovatt S, Myint PK, Loke YK. Misdiagnosis of pulmonary embolism and missed pulmonary embolism: A systematic review of the literature. Health Sciences Review. 2022;**3**:100022

[15] Howard L. Acute pulmonary embolism. Clinical Medicine. 2019;**19**(3):243

[16] Konstantinides SV, Barco S, Lankeit M, Meyer G. Management of

pulmonary embolism: An update.
Journal of the American College of
Cardiology. 2016;**67**(8):976-990

[17] Kuo WT, Van Den Bosch MA,
Hofmann LV, Louie JD, Kothary N,
Sze DY. Catheter-directed embolectomy,
fragmentation, and thrombolysis for the
treatment of massive pulmonary
embolism after failure of systemic
thrombolysis. Chest. 2008;**134**(2):
250-254

[18] Gulba DC, Lichtlen P, Schmid C,
Borst H, Dietz R, Luft F. Medical
compared with surgical treatment for
massive pulmonary embolism. The
Lancet. 1994;**343**(8897):576-577

Chapter 2

Diagnosis of Pulmonary Embolism

Sachin M. Patil

Abstract

Pulmonary embolism is an acute emergency due to the occlusion of the pulmonary arteries by a venous blood clot. The pathophysiology of pulmonary embolism follows Virchow's triad, which encompasses stasis in veins, increased coagulation, and vessel wall trauma. Pregnancy, major trauma or surgery, prolonged immobilization, obesity, medication, and inherited risks are important risks. It is an essential rule-out diagnosis in chest pain and dyspnea patients in the emergency room. It is also responsible for significant mortality if not diagnosed and treated promptly. Physicians utilize multiple algorithmic scores and calculators to supplement diagnosis along with a high degree of clinical suspicion at initial presentation. Clinical diagnosis involves utilizing multiple modalities, including D-dimer, troponin, arterial blood gas analysis, electrocardiogram, bedside echocardiogram, and imaging modalities such as venous duplex, chest computed tomography, ventilation-perfusion scans, and pulmonary angiogram. Some imaging modalities carry the risk of radiation and being invasive. The treatment can itself be short-term or lifelong based on the causative factor. Anticoagulants used in the therapy can itself cause devastating complications if not monitored appropriately. Despite adequate treatment, some of these patients progress to chronic disease resulting in secondary pulmonary hypertension.

Keywords: Pulmonary embolism, diagnosis, computed tomography, risk factors

1. Introduction

Acute Pulmonary embolism (PE) is an emergency. It needs immediate clinical evaluation for appropriate recognition due to the availability of appropriate therapeutic interventions to decrease its immediate mortality and avoid postthrombotic complications. Clinical manifestations of a patient coupled with the risk factors at initial presentation should guide to PE suspicion. In cases where the clinical scenario is not straightforward, multiple algorithmic score models should promptly guide the physician to diagnose PE. PE diagnosis is accomplished with the help of multiple imaging studies, of which chest computed tomography (CT) is the one used frequently. In this topic, we will glean over all the factors that help in diagnosing an acute PE.

2. Epidemiology

Acute pulmonary embolism (PE) is an acute critical clinical condition characterized by the propagation of blood clots from peripheral veins or systemic circulation to the lung vasculature affecting the alveolar gas exchange. Acute PE can be symptomatic or silent. The thrombus responsible for PE often originates from leg veins, especially the deep calf veins, followed by proximal dispersion to popliteal and femoral veins [1]. Thrombus at popliteal vein and proximal to it are at a high risk of embolic phenomenon resulting in acute PE. A non-propagating deep calf vein thrombus increases recurrence rate and the likelihood of postphlebitic complication [2]. A thrombus from the upper extremity is often due to intravascular venous catheters, cardiac devices, effort thrombosis, or thoracic outlet obstruction [3]. Pelvic veins represent another source of emboli in patients with recent pelvic surgery, pregnancy, infection, or prostate disease. Rarely pulmonary vascular occlusion occurs due to nonthrombus etiology such as parasites (schistosomiasis), sickled erythrocytes (sickle cell disease), talc (illicit drugs), air (central lines), or tissue (amniotic fluid or fat embolism).

Earlier clinical literature suggested PE as an underdiagnosed condition; however, recent studies indicate it to be an excessively diagnosed condition due to the introduction of modern imaging techniques in detecting PE [4, 5]. Newer studies indicate an increased incidence at >113 cases per 100,000 population [5]. Another reason is defensive medicine, as the inability to identify a clinically symptomatic patient could turn out to be a malpractice issue as only 8% die with appropriate therapy, and the figure is 30% with no therapy [6–8]. Even with an increased incidence, the overall mortality rate has remained the same, declining case fatality rates [5]. The DVT/PE incidence rate in the United States of America (USA) yearly is 600,000 patients per year [9]. Approximately 30% of these patients die within the next 3 months (180,000 per year) [4]. In medical or surgical intensive care units (MICU/SICU), deep vein thrombosis (DVT) occurs in 30% of patients [10, 11]. In an extensive registry of diagnosed DVT patients, PE was seen in 29% in the lower extremity(LE) and 9% in the arms [12]. PE occurrence was similar in these groups on observing them over the next 90 days. PE is a frequent preventable mortality source in hospitalized patients [13]. Despite anticoagulant therapy in critically ill, acute PE is linked with considerable morbidity and mortality due to a limited cardiopulmonary reserve [14]. After the acute critical episode, patients who make it out are at higher risk of type four pulmonary hypertension and postthrombotic syndrome. A recent study confirms that after 6 months of a PE episode, dissolution of the entire clot was observed in 50% of patients, and the remaining still had lingering occlusion [15, 16].

3. Clinical features

Symptomatic patients with acute respiratory failure should increase diagnostic possibility if they have risk elements. These risk factors have been mentioned in **Table 1** [1, 13, 14].

Clinical features depend on the patient's physiologic response to the venous thrombus, especially cardiopulmonary reserve, and vary from asymptomatic to hemodynamic instability and death. An excellent clinical history can reveal risks, including hormone replacement therapy, bed rest, air or road travel, oral contraceptive use, and other comorbid conditions. Clinical symptoms include acute respiratory distress (most common), chest discomfort, dry cough, fever, leg swelling with or without pain, bloody expectoration, and rarely syncopal episode. The physical examination can reveal tachycardia, tachypnea, hypotension, phlebitis, rales, a loud P2, and an S4. It may also reveal other signs indicative of risk factors. Of the above clinical features, only three can distinguish between positive and negative PE based on angiogram, including rales, a loud P2, and S4 [17]. Clinical presentation to a hospital is seen via five different syndromes, which include 1) Pleuritic chest discomfort or bloody

Acquired	Inherited
A. **Immobilization**	1. Factor V Leiden mutation
Bed rest due to hospitalization or stroke	2. Prothrombin gene mutation
Air travel	3. Antithrombin III deficiency
Post-operative: Hip/Knee/Trauma/Spinal	4. Protein C deficiency
Morbid Obesity	5. Protein S deficiency
Comorbidities: Heart failure, Obstructive lung disease, elderly, prior stroke	6. Dysfibrinogenemia
B. **Procoagulant Hormonal conditions**	
Pregnancy/Postpartum	
Oral contraceptives	
Hormonal replacement therapy	
C. **Hematological conditions**	
Polycythemia vera, Essential thrombocytosis	
Leukemia, Paroxysmal Nocturnal Hemoglobinuria	
Antiphospholipid antibody syndrome	
D. **Others**	
Nephrotic syndrome, Inflammatory Bowel disease	
Malignancy	

Table 1.
Risk factors for DVT/PE.

expectoration, 2) Shortness of breath only, 3) Hemodynamic instability, 4) Subclinical clot, 5) Chronic non-resolving clot [1, 17]. The fourth and fifth clinical syndrome may be identified incidentally on the imaging studies while working for dyspnea of unknown origin or as a study to rule out other clinical conditions.

4. Non-imaging modalities

A complete blood cell count can disclose leukocytosis, while a peripheral smear and a differential count can reveal leukemia, myeloproliferative disorders, or other hematological conditions. NLR (Neutrophil to lymphocyte ratio) and PLR (platelet to lymphocyte ratio) if elevated at PE diagnosis signify an elevated short-term risk and overall mortality; however, the exact cutoff for NLR and PLR is yet to be decided. Both NLR and PLR can serve as cheap prognostic indicators in acute PE [18]. Acute PE causes myocardial distension and stretching, leading to an increase in BNP (Brain Natriuretic Peptide) and NT-proBNP (N-terminal pro-brain Natriuretic Peptide). The right ventricle (RV) undergoes significant strain during an acute massive PE, resulting in RV ischemia that can be small and cause elevated troponin and H-FABP (heart-type fatty acid-binding protein levels). Elevated above-mentioned cardiac biomarkers and troponin in nonmassive PE signify higher short-term mortality and PE-related adverse events [19, 20]. Also, in nonmassive PE, RV dysfunction correlated appropriately with short-term mortality [20]. Arterial blood gases (ABG) reveal hypoxemia in acute PE, which can worsen with increased PE size. PE leads to increased dead space ventilation and hypercapnia; however, this is seen in patients with limited ventilatory reserve or mechanically ventilated patients [1]. In an earlier study, a 100% NPV (negative predictive value) for PE correlated with respiratory rate < 20 per minute, normal D-dimer level, and partial pressure of oxygen ≥80 mmHg [21]. This was later found to have an NPV of 95% in a more extensive study where multiple ABG prediction rules were assessed and were found to lack adequate NPV, likelihood ratios, or specificity [22]. Thus ABG has minimal conclusive value in suspected PE patients and is inadequate to diagnose or exclude PE.

D-dimer presence in blood indicates intrinsic fibrinolysis by plasmin. In DVT, D-dimer elevation is lesser than that seen in PE due to the smaller size of the thrombus. Thus D-dimer sensitivity is higher in PE (> 95%) than in DVT (>80%) [13]. The D-dimer elevation is observed in infection, inflammation, ischemia, cancer, trauma, and postoperatively making it a nonspecific test. Thus its predictive role in hospitalized patients is minimal. D-dimer is outstanding in patients <65 years of age plus lower pretest PE probability. D-dimer had a diminishing value in the patient subset >65 years of age due to more false positives [23]. Another study suggested using age-adjusted D-dimer testing alongside Well's score as it improved efficiency with no effect on safety in all subgroups studied. The efficiency was notably observed in elderly patients, patients with cancer, obstructive lung disease, prior venous thromboembolism, or a late presentation [24]. A standardized hypersensitive negative test result safely rules out PE among mild or moderate-risk patients [1].

In a small proportion(10–25%) of PE patients an ECG (electrocardiogram) is normal [25]. ECG can reveal multiple findings that lack sensitivity and specificity individually to diagnose PE. The commonest ECG finding is acute sinus tachycardia [26]. Other significant ECG findings are mentioned in **Table 2** below [27].

In an established extensive PE, a frequent earlier finding is precordial T wave inversions [28]. The observation of S1Q3T3, RBBB, and inverted T waves (V1-V4 leads) in a PE patient's ECG indicated RV dysfunction [28, 29]. V1 to V3 precordial lead T wave inversions had a higher true positive rate and diagnostic accuracy than S1Q3T3 and RBBB findings in RV dysfunction detection in acute PE [30]. If ECG reveals an RV strain pattern, the patient is at a higher mortality risk and adverse outcomes, despite being hemodynamically stable [31]. RBBB, Lead V1 ST-segment elevation, and low voltage QRS complexes are observed in PE patients with cardiogenic shock [32]. The following findings were frequently seen in patients who had a fatal outcome after a PE, including complete RBBB, atrial arrhythmias, Q wave (leads III & aVF), Peripheral small amplitudes, and left precordial ST changes. In a study, 29% of patients with these ECG findings did not make it out of the hospital on discharge [33]. A concurrent occurrence of inverted T waves in leads II, III, aVF, and V1 to V4 is highly distinct for PE (99%) than ACS but uncommon [34]. Acute PE accurately

1. Acute sinus tachycardia
2. T wave inversions in precordial leads (V1-V4)
3. S1Q3T3 sign (Lead I S wave, Lead III Q wave, and a Lead III inverted T wave)
4. Atrial arrhythmias
5. RBBB (Right bundle branch block)
6. Low amplitude QRS complexes
7. ST-segment elevation in leads V1 and aVR
8. Q wave (Leads III and aVF)

Table 2.
ECG findings in acute PE.

distinguishes from ACS by the presence of lead III and V1 T wave inversions on ECG [35]. An essential role of performing an EKG in acute PE is its help in ruling out other differential diagnoses, such as ACS, myocarditis, or acute pericarditis.

5. Noninvasive imaging modalities

Venous duplex ultrasound uses the ability to detect venous blood flow and real-time B-mode images to identify clots in both upper and lower limbs [36]. The specific diagnostic DVT criteria include the following, lack of venous segment collapse on pressure (more specific), respiration induced loss of phase changes, a weak venous response to Valsalva, echogenic substance in the lumen, loss of increase in flow due to compression, and loss of flow or decreased flow on color Doppler [1]. In symptomatic patients, duplex ultrasonography sensitivity and specificity in diagnosing DVT are higher than in asymptomatic patients (lesser accuracy). While 30–40% of PE patients are clinically symptomatic for proximal DVT, the venous duplex can detect proximal DVT in 60–80% of PE patients [37]. In postoperative orthopedic patients, the performance of venous duplex ultrasound was comparable to contrast venography in asymptomatic proximal DVT detection [38]. Asymptomatic DVT in contralateral LE was seen in 5–10% of patients with acute symptomatic DVT [39]. Duplex ultrasonography accuracy in identifying deep calf vein limited DVT, and asymptomatic proximal vein DVT is limited in high-risk populations [40]. After an initially negative result in suspected DVT patients, serial duplex ultrasonography can detect the proximal extension [41].

The sensitivity of detecting PE via TTE (transthoracic echocardiogram) is only 50%, so it is a poor imaging modality for acute PE diagnosis [42]. RV pressure or volume overload suggestive of PE can guide PE diagnostic imaging without other differentials [1]. TTE can reveal the McConnell sign (RV mid-free wall lack of movement with no apex involvement) [43]. On rare occasions, emboli can be visualized in the right heart on TTE. TTE based risk assessment helps in guiding acute PE therapy. Patients with RV dysfunction on TTE in a normotensive patient indicate adverse outcomes or early mortality [44, 45]. An appropriately done TEE (transesophageal echocardiogram) can detect central PE (Pulmonary artery and its branches) with a true positive and negative rate > 90% [46]. It is an excellent modality to consider in a speculated massive PE patient hemodynamically unstable for transport or has contrast contraindication. TTE helps ward off other differential diagnoses, including infective endocarditis, pericardial effusion or tamponade, aortic dissection, and RV myocardial infarction. Significant changes seen on a TTE are mentioned below in **Table 3** [47].

A meta-analysis assessed multiple echo studies and consistently showed that TTE had a greater specificity and sensitivity for PE diagnosis and is a definitive rule in test at the bedside for suspected patients [47]. As per ACEP guidelines, the presence of an RV dysfunction on TTE in an unstable patient can suggest acute PE and an indication for thrombolytic therapy [48].

A positive or negative transthoracic lung ultrasound (TLS) can cause an increment or decrement in PE probability by 30% in a moderate risk population, which can change the diagnostic workup [49]. TLS can detect smaller PE in the periphery of the lungs [50]. Most emboli are observed in the lower lungs, which can be easily accessed by TLS [51]. An endobronchial ultrasound (EBUS) can detect central PE and immensely help PE patients with AKI, contrast contraindication, pregnancy, and hemodynamically unstable patients with diagnosis [52–54]. Simultaneously it can measure the acutely elevated pulmonary hypertension in patients with PE. Endobronchial ultrasound findings can supplement TLS in acute PE detection [49].

1. Increased ventricle size ratio	
2. Abnormal septal motion	
3. Tricuspid valve regurgitation (TVR)	
4. 60/60 sign	
5. McConnell's sign	
6. Right heart thrombus	
7. Right ventricle hypokinesis	
8. Pulmonary hypertension	
9. Increased right ventricle end-diastolic diameter (RVEDD)	
10. Tricuspid annular plane systolic excursion (TAPSE)	
11. Increased right ventricle systolic pressure (RVSP)	

Table 3.
Distinct TTE signs seen in acute PE.

However, the resources required (regular bronchoscope, trained nursing staff) to perform a bedside bronchoscopy with EBUS makes it challenging to achieve in the emergency department or the MICU on an as-needed basis. Performing a bronchoscopy in a hemodynamically unstable patient may worsen the patient's overall cardiopulmonary status and increase his high risk of adverse outcomes.

A meta-analysis revealed that cardiopulmonary ultrasound (CPUS) sensitivity was 91% and specificity was 81% for PE diagnosis in comparison to CT pulmonary angiography (CTPA) [55]. The BLUE (bedside lung ultrasound in emergency) protocol was made to diagnose PE based on a DVT positive venous duplex combined with TLS. It was 99% specific and 81% sensitive for PE diagnosis and ruled out other acute respiratory failure differentials [56]. BLUE protocol and TTE consistently revealed a greater specificity than sensitivity due to the lack of ruling PE out with no CTPA [56, 57]. The combination may help in decreasing the excessive CTPA done currently [58]. In resource-limited settings such as in developing countries or the absence of CTPA availability, CPUS may have a role in managing PE [55].

Chest X-ray can either be normal or abnormal. Most often, a chest X-ray reveals nonspecific abnormal findings such as effusion, infiltrates, or atelectasis. Certain signs with interesting names that have been observed on chest radiograph imaging are mentioned in **Table 4** [59–61].

The occurrence of Westermark's sign and Palla's sign suggests embolic obstruction of either the lobar/segmental pulmonary artery/widespread small arterial involvement [60]. A patient with acute shortness of breath, respiratory distress, or hypoxia and a benign chest radiograph is suspicious of possible PE. A chest radiograph also helps in ruling out other causes such as empyema, pneumonia, and pneumothorax.

1. Westermark's sign	Localized diminished blood supply in lung
2. Hampton's hump	Pulmonary infarction distal to occluded emboli (Wedge shape)
3. Palla's sign	Distended right descending pulmonary artery or sausage appearance
4. Fleischner sign	Central pulmonary enlargement
5. Knuckle sign	Abrupt pulmonary artery tapering

Table 4.
Interesting findings noted on chest-X-ray.

After CTPA, V/Q (ventilation/perfusion) scintigraphy is an alternative utilized in diagnosis. V/Q scintigraphy negative or high-probability result is of critical value in PE diagnosis [62, 63]. A negative V/Q scan result is as efficacious as a pulmonary angiogram, ruling out acute PE and slightly better than a CTPA [64]. A normal perfusion scan sensitivity in ruling out PE is exceptional, observed even with a higher pretest PE probability in severely sick patients [62, 65, 66]. A meta-analysis validates this observation by revealing a minimal 0.3% PE incidence in individuals with an intact perfusion result [67]. Similarly, high-risk V/Q scintigraphy (multi-segmental mismatch defects) correlates with acute PE in 87% of patients, and the positive predictive value (PPV) is increased to 96% by a higher pretest probability [62]. However, most suspected acute PE or PE patients do not have V/Q scan findings suggestive of a high probability scan. Also, most patients with no PE did not have a normal V/Q result. A clinically significant portion of patients (33% = moderate risk and 10% = low risk) had positive angiograms. The prospective trial PIOPED stressed on the number of perfusion defects and size along with a concurrent image to identify V/Q mismatch defects [62]. In the PISA-PED study, greater emphasis was placed on the perfusion defect shape than the number and size or ventilation image correlation [65]. The PISA-PED study confirmed that perfusion in combination with pretest probability in the absence of ventilation image could diagnose acute PE without angiography [65]. A majority of intermediate V/Q imaging results are observed in obstructive lung disease patients [68]. V/Q scintigraphy is favored in patients with renal failure, contrast allergy and offers similar diagnostic efficacy in pregnancy [1, 69]. The severely sick patients can undergo bedside perfusion imaging to avoid transportation-associated risks [1].

SPECT-V/Q scan, a new scintigraphy process that generates 3-dimensional images than a planar image seen in V/Q scans. Advantages associated are better visualization of all perfusion defects in different lung areas, less radiation exposure than CTPA, fewer nondiagnostic test results (0.5–3%) [70–75]. SPECT-V/Q efficiency is similar to that of CTPA in suspected acute PE patients [76]. SPECT-V/Q true positive and negative rates were noted to be in the range of 95–100% [76, 77]. However, it cannot replace CTPA as a test of choice in acute PE due to the lack of vigorous extensive testing to verify its validity in suspected patients [78]. Specific clinical scenarios might be appropriate for using a SPECT-VQ scan, including a nondiagnostic CTPA study and post-discharge evaluation of lingering perfusion abnormalities.

The imaging modality of choice to exclude acute PE in suspected patients is CTPA. CTPA sensitivity is 83%, specificity is 96%, with an NPV of 97% plus a PPV of 86% in suspected patients [17]. CTPA sensitivity and specificity are greater than 95% in central PE (pulmonary artery and lobar branches) [79]. The sensitivity and specificity decline gradually when the emboli involve segmental or subsegmental pulmonary arteries. In a study of CTPA for subsegmental artery, involvement sensitivity was noted in the range of 71–84% [80]. PE involving only the subsegmental arteries of the pulmonary circulation is seen in around 30% of PE patients [81, 82]. CTPA evaluation is diagnostic when emboli involve the main or lobar pulmonary arteries and is considered suggestive if the segmental and subsegmental pulmonary arteries are occluded. CTPA predictive value is critically hampered in discordance with clinical evaluation, and further imaging tests merit consideration in this scenario [1]. CTPA has its limitations which are significant to be ignored. Intravenous iodinated contrast given during CTPA can cause AKI. CTPA cannot effectively diagnose emboli in the subsegmental pulmonary arteries and cannot supplement the V/Q scan, which also lacks in this particular territory [62, 81]. CTPA is not able to identify whether the emboli is acute, subacute, or chronic. CTPA occurrence results in significant radiation exposure to the patient, especially in young females (breast and lungs) [83]. Clinical observations have suggested significant overuse of CTPA resulting in overdiagnosis of pulmonary embolism; however, it cannot determine whether the positive CTPA identifies acute PE, subacute PE, or chronic PE [63]. A clinical study observed no substantial difference in results when anticoagulation was withheld in suspected individuals with a normal CTPA plus negative leg duplex ultrasonography and negative or non-high probable V/Q imaging with a negative leg venous duplex [63]. The study was performed on relatively stable patients, so this observation cannot be utilized in severely sick patients or patients with inadequate cardiopulmonary reserve [84].

A clinical trial PIOPED III evaluated a magnetic resonance angiogram for PE diagnosis [85]. Overall, the sensitivity to diagnose a PE involving the main and lobar pulmonary artery was 79%. It may be an ideal test for patients with intravenous contrast allergy or to avoid radiation exposure, such as pregnancy.

6. Invasive imaging modalities

CT venography (CTV) has similar diagnostic accuracy as venous duplex ultrasound for the LE in diagnosing or ruling out DVT; however, the test is invasive and comes with exposure to contrast and radiation [86]. In addition to the LE venous system, vena cava and pelvic veins are visualized. CTPA and CTV combined revealed a mild improvement in diagnostic outcome with a substantial increase in cost and pelvic exposure to radiation.

Contrast venography is the best imaging study for substantiating LE venous thrombosis. Its diagnostic criteria include a persistent venous filling defect observed in ≥ two views. It is an expensive, invasive test requiring clinical expertise and accurate interpretation with significant exposure to intravenous iodine contrast. Due to the above reasons, Venous duplex has replaced it as the test of choice to diagnose acute DVT.

Before CTPA, a pulmonary angiogram was the best imaging study to diagnose acute PE. It requires appropriate clinical expertise to perform the invasive procedure and interpret it. Three factors determine the result, including the location of the emboli, image quality, and interpreter's experience [1]. Diagnosis of PE is indicated by either a filling defect and/or abrupt vessel cutoff. Flow defects can be avoided by ensuring good vascular opacification and obtaining multiple sequences of films. The PIOPED trial revealed that it was diagnostic in 97% of patients and associated with 1% complications, including a mortality rate of 0.5% [87]. Adverse outcomes were significantly seen in MICU patients transported for an angiogram. A pulmonary angiogram is considered in a tiny patient subset when PE diagnosis cannot be determined by noninvasive imaging studies, significant discordance between imaging study and clinical evaluation, and chronic thromboembolic disease.

7. Diagnostic workup

The current clinical approach for acute PE or DVT diagnosis utilizes a Bayesian analysis. Here pretest probability of the clinical condition is measured exclusive of the test outcome wire clinical means or a consistent prediction rule such as Well's or Geneva score. Then a posttest probability of the clinical condition is generated by utilizing pretest probability combined with a test's likelihood ratio. The posttest probability is used as guidance for clinical decision making that confirms or to excludes the disease with a degree of probability or helps in deciding additional imaging studies. Clinical predictive rules for acute DVT include the Well's, revised Well's, and Geneva scores. Well's score classifies suspected acute DVT patients into three subclassification's unlikely (3%), moderate (17%), and likely (75%). With the help of Well's score

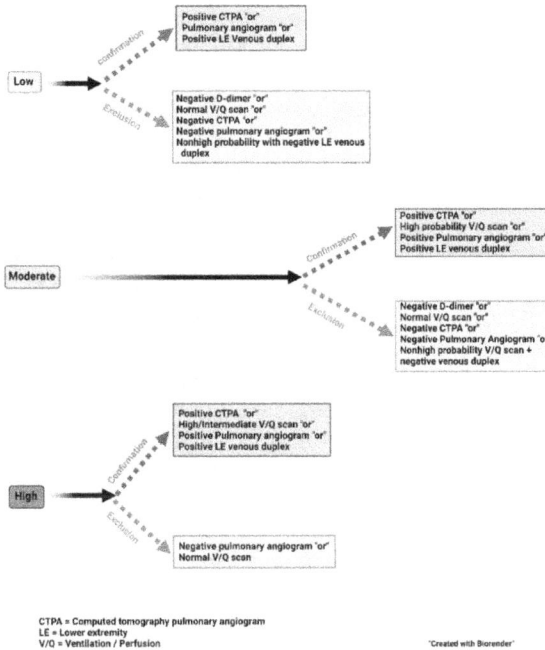

Figure 1.
Diagnostic testing of acute PE based on clinical probability.

and LE venous duplex ultrasound, diagnosis of acute DVT can be established in likely individuals with a positive LE venous duplex result. In unlikely individuals, a negative LE venous duplex result excludes acute DVT [88]. The revised Well's score divided the patients into likely and unlikely categories. The unlikely group with a negative D-dimer excluded an acute DVT without needing a LE venous duplex ultrasound [89, 90].

Clinical predictive tools for acute PE include Well's criteria, revised Geneva score, Pisa model, PERC (PE rule-out criteria), and Charlotte rule [91–95]. Among the clinical predictor rules or scores for acute PE diagnosis, Well's score fared better than the revised Geneva score [96]. Most diagnostic algorithms for acute PE use either CTPA or V/Q scintigraphy as a first test. A diagnostic algorithm based on clinical probability has been described in **Figure 1** below for acute PE.

Clinical predictive rules or scores are not superior to clinical assessment but offset the variation observed with physician judgment and experience by standardization [1]. These rules were framed for patients seen in outpatient settings and applicable in primary care and emergency departments; however, they fare poorly and lack clinical validity in hospitalized patients. In hospitalized patients, the clinical predictive scores or rules and D-dimer are of minimal help to make a clinical decision. As a result, most of these patients need an imaging study to rule in or exclude acute PE diagnosis [1].

8. COVID-19 infection and venous thromboembolism

Although acutely ill patients are at a higher risk of acute PE, COVID -19 (coronavirus disease 2019) infected patients suffer from in situ immunothrombosis characterized by small and medium pulmonary artery numerous thrombi occurring at a greater frequency (24%) than in H1N1 influenza patients [97–101]. PE phenotype in COVID-19 patients in comparison to others correlates with peripheral thrombotic lesions with a lesser clot burden [102]. Pulmonary localized immunothrombosis in COVID-19 is a minimal addition to the overall procoagulant state resulting in DVT seen only in 42.4% of PE patients in COVID-19 than the 60% occurrence seen frequently in other PE patients [103]. D-dimer elevation in COVID-19 could be due to the acute infection-induced inflammation causing a procoagulant state or a localized micro thrombosis in the pulmonary vasculature.

D-dimer levels elevation >500 µg/L & 1000 µg/L were associated with a higher sensitivity (> 90%) but a lower specificity (< 30%) in PE diagnosis. D-dimer performance in COVID-19 is similar to that seen in other prothrombotic conditions [104]. COVID-19 patients on statin therapy before admission had a lower risk of PE occurrence [105]. COVID-19 patients with significant inflammation measured by elevated C-reactive protein and D-dimer were at a higher risk of acute PE [106]. PE was detected frequently in the periphery than in the central pulmonary arteries [107]. The most frequent site was the segmental, followed by the lobar, central, and subsegmental PE [106]. Acute PE was observed at a greater prevalence in COVID-19 patients with an increased Body mass index (BMI) [106].

A systematic review and meta-analysis on PE and DVT in COVID-19 patients disclosed a higher pooled PE incidence of 24.7% in ICU patients. This percentage is substantially higher than the proportion seen in other viral pneumonia admitted to ICU in the presence or absence of acute respiratory distress syndrome (1.3%–7.5%) [108, 109]. In contrast, it was 10.5% in non-ICU patients (higher than the usual) [107]. Overall the incidence rates of PE and DVT in COVID-19 patients were 16.5% and 14.8% [107]. COVID -19 infection severity and CTPA universal screening correlated with a greater frequency of PE diagnosis. DVT was a concurrent finding in 42.4% of patients with acute PE. An elevated BMI (> 30) correlated substantially with a 2.7 times higher frequency of an acute PE [106]. As observed in a recent study, obese patients with COVID-19 suffer from a more severe disease [110]. A meta-analysis revealed an increased prevalence of venous thromboembolism and acute PE with increasing age in COVID-19 patients [111].

9. Conclusion

Acute PE is an emergency, and ongoing research will reveal newer biochemical assays and better imaging studies for accurate earlier detection of acute PE in the upcoming few years. SPECT V/Q scan is currently undergoing evaluation at multiple centers where it is being compared to planar V/Q study and CTPA in suspected PE patients for accuracy. Physicians must understand the fallacies of each biochemical test and imaging study for their appropriate utilization in a clinical scenario for the patient's best outcome. Critical ECG findings and bedside echocardiogram findings should be stressed upon admission and utilized for prognostification. Physicians should be aware that these clinical scores or prediction rules play no role in hospitalized patients and should not be used for decision-making in this particular patient subset.

Acknowledgements

"No external funds have been utilized in the preparation of this manuscript."

Conflict of interest

"We declare no conflict of interest."

Notes/thanks/other declarations

"We thank the editor for allowing us to author this manuscript.

Acronyms and abbreviations

PE	Pulmonary embolism
CT	Computed tomography
USA	United States of America
MICU	Medical intensive care unit
SICU	Surgical intensive care unit
DVT	Deep vein thrombosis
LE	Lower extremity
P2	Pulmonic component of second heart sound
S4	Fourth heart sound
NLR	Neutrophil to Lymphocyte ratio
PLR	Platelet to Lymphocyte ratio
NT-proBNP	N-terminal pro Brain natriuretic peptide
BNP	Brain natriuretic peptide
RV	Right ventricle
H-FABP	Heart-type fatty acid-binding protein
ABG	Arterial blood gas
NPV	Negative predictive value
ECG	Electrocardiogram
RBBB	Right bundle branch block
ACS	Acute coronary syndrome
TTE	Transthoracic echocardiogram
TEE	Transesophageal echocardiogram
TVR	Tricuspid valve regurgitation
RVEDD	Right ventricle end-diastolic diameter
TAPSE	Tricuspid annular plane systolic excursion
RVSP	Right ventricle systolic pressure
ACEP	American College of Emergency physicians
TLS	Transthoracic lung ultrasound
EBUS	Endobronchial ultrasound
CPUS	Cardiopulmonary ultrasound
CTPA	Computed tomography pulmonary angiography
BLUE	Bedside lung ultrasound in emergency
V/Q	Ventilation / Perfusion
PIOPED	Prospective investigation of pulmonary embolism diagnosis
PISA-PED	Prospective Investigative Study of Acute Pulmonary Embolism

Diagnosis

SPECT	Single Photon Emission Computed Tomography
CTV	Computed tomography venography
PERC	Pulmonary embolism rule-out criteria
COVID-19	Coronavirus disease 2019
BMI	Body mass index

Author details

Sachin M. Patil
Infectious Disease Critical Care, University of Missouri, Columbia, MO, USA

*Address all correspondence to: drssmp1@gmail.com

IntechOpen

References

[1] Fedullo PF, Yung GL. Pulmonary thromboembolic disease. In: Grippi MA, Elias JA, Fishman JA, Kotloff RM, Pack AI, Senior RM, et al., editors. Fishman's Pulmonary Diseases and Disorders. 5e ed. New York, NY: McGraw-Hill Education; 2015

[2] Masuda EM, Kistner RL, Musikasinthorn C, Liquido F, Geling O, He Q. The controversy of managing calf vein thrombosis. Journal of Vascular Surgery. 2012;**55**(2):550-561

[3] Mai C, Hunt D. Upper-extremity deep venous thrombosis: A review. The American Journal of Medicine. 2011;**124**(5):402-407

[4] Heit JA, Silverstein MD, Mohr DN, Petterson TM, O'Fallon WM, Melton LJ 3rd. Predictors of survival after deep vein thrombosis and pulmonary embolism: A population-based, cohort study. Archives of Internal Medicine. 1999;**159**(5):445-453

[5] Wiener RS, Schwartz LM, Woloshin S. Time trends in pulmonary embolism in the United States: evidence of overdiagnosis. Archives of Internal Medicine. 2011;**171**(9):831-837

[6] Dalen JE, Alpert JS. Natural history of pulmonary embolism. Progress in Cardiovascular Diseases. 1975;**17**(4): 259-270

[7] Hermann RE, Davis JH, Holden WD, Pulmonary embolism. A clinical and pathologic study with emphasis on the effect of prophylactic therapy with anticoagulants. American Journal of Surgery. 1961;**102**:19-28

[8] Byrne JJ. Phlebitis; a study of 748 cases at the Boston City Hospital. The New England Journal of Medicine. 1955;**253**(14):579-586

[9] Anderson FA Jr, Wheeler HB, Goldberg RJ, Hosmer DW, Patwardhan NA, Jovanovic B, et al. A population-based perspective of the hospital incidence and case-fatality rates of deep vein thrombosis and pulmonary embolism. The Worcester DVT Study. Archives of Internal Medicine. 1991;**151**(5):933-938

[10] Attia J, Ray JG, Cook DJ, Douketis J, Ginsberg JS, Geerts WH. Deep vein thrombosis and its prevention in critically ill adults. Archives of Internal Medicine. 2001;**161**(10):1268-1279

[11] Hirsch DR, Ingenito EP, Goldhaber SZ. Prevalence of deep venous thrombosis among patients in medical intensive care. JAMA. 1995;**274**(4):335-337

[12] Munoz FJ, Mismetti P, Poggio R, Valle R, Barron M, Guil M, et al. Clinical outcome of patients with upper-extremity deep vein thrombosis: results from the RIETE Registry. Chest. 2008;**133**(1):143-148

[13] Goldhaber SZ. Deep Venous Thrombosis and Pulmonary Thromboembolism. In: Jameson JL, Fauci AS, Kasper DL, Hauser SL, Longo DL, Loscalzo J, editors. Harrison's Principles of Internal Medicine. 20e ed. New York, NY: McGraw-Hill Education; 2018

[14] Meyer NJ, Schmidt GA. Pulmonary Embolic Disorders: Thrombus, Air, and Fat. In: Hall JB, Schmidt GA, Kress JP, editors. Principles of Critical Care. 4e ed. New York, NY: McGraw-Hill Education; 2015

[15] Nijkeuter M, Hovens MM, Davidson BL, Huisman MV. Resolution of thromboemboli in patients with acute pulmonary embolism: A systematic review. Chest. 2006;**129**(1):192-197

[16] Wartski M, Collignon MA. Incomplete recovery of lung perfusion

after 3 months in patients with acute pulmonary embolism treated with antithrombotic agents. THESEE Study Group. Tinzaparin ou Heparin Standard: Evaluation dans l'Embolie Pulmonaire Study. Journal of Nuclear Medicine. 2000;**41**(6):1043-1048

[17] Stein PD, Beemath A, Matta F, Weg JG, Yusen RD, Hales CA, et al. Clinical characteristics of patients with acute pulmonary embolism: Data from PIOPED II. The American Journal of Medicine. 2007;**120**(10):871-879

[18] Wang Q, Ma J, Jiang Z, Ming L. Prognostic value of neutrophil-to-lymphocyte ratio and platelet-to-lymphocyte ratio in acute pulmonary embolism: A systematic review and meta-analysis. International Angiology. 2018;**37**(1):4-11

[19] Bajaj A, Rathor P, Sehgal V, Kabak B, Shetty A, Al Masalmeh O, et al. Prognostic Value of Biomarkers in Acute Non-massive Pulmonary Embolism: A Systematic Review and Meta-analysis. Lung. 2015;**193**(5):639-651

[20] Barco S, Mahmoudpour SH, Planquette B, Sanchez O, Konstantinides SV, Meyer G. Prognostic value of right ventricular dysfunction or elevated cardiac biomarkers in patients with low-risk pulmonary embolism: A systematic review and meta-analysis. European Heart Journal. 2019;**40**(11): 902-910

[21] Egermayer P, Town GI, Turner JG, Heaton DC, Mee AL, Beard ME. Usefulness of D-dimer, blood gas, and respiratory rate measurements for excluding pulmonary embolism. Thorax. 1998;**53**(10):830-834

[22] Rodger MA, Carrier M, Jones GN, Rasuli P, Raymond F, Djunaedi H, et al. Diagnostic value of arterial blood gas measurement in suspected pulmonary embolism. American Journal of Respiratory and Critical Care Medicine. 2000;**162**(6):2105-2108

[23] Crawford F, Andras A, Welch K, Sheares K, Keeling D, Chappell FM. D-dimer test for excluding the diagnosis of pulmonary embolism. Cochrane Database of Systematic Reviews. 2016;**8**:CD010864

[24] van Es N, van der Hulle T, van Es J, den Exter PL, Douma RA, Goekoop RJ, et al. Wells Rule and d-Dimer Testing to Rule Out Pulmonary Embolism: A Systematic Review and Individual-Patient Data Meta-analysis. Annals of Internal Medicine. 2016;**165**(4):253-261

[25] Hubloue I, Schoors D, Diltoer M, Van Tussenbroek F, de Wilde P. Early electrocardiographic signs in acute massive pulmonary embolism. European Journal of Emergency Medicine. 1996;**3**(3):199-204

[26] Petruzzelli S, Palla A, Pieraccini F, Donnamaria V, Giuntini C. Routine electrocardiography in screening for pulmonary embolism. Respiration. 1986;**50**(4):233-243

[27] Chan TC, Vilke GM, Pollack M, Brady WJ. Electrocardiographic manifestations: Pulmonary embolism. The Journal of Emergency Medicine. 2001;**21**(3):263-270

[28] Ferrari E, Imbert A, Chevalier T, Mihoubi A, Morand P, Baudouy M. The ECG in pulmonary embolism. Predictive value of negative T waves in precordial leads--80 case reports. Chest. 1997; **111**(3):537-543

[29] Daniel KR, Courtney DM, Kline JA. Assessment of cardiac stress from massive pulmonary embolism with 12-lead ECG. Chest. 2001;**120**(2):474-481

[30] Punukollu G, Gowda RM, Vasavada BC, Khan IA. Role of electrocardiography in identifying right ventricular dysfunction in acute pulmonary embolism. The American Journal of Cardiology. 2005;**96**(3):450-452

[31] Vanni S, Polidori G, Vergara R, Pepe G, Nazerian P, Moroni F, et al. Prognostic value of ECG among patients with acute pulmonary embolism and normal blood pressure. The American Journal of Medicine. 2009;**122**(3):257-264

[32] Kukla P, McIntyre WF, Fijorek K, Mirek-Bryniarska E, Bryniarski L, Krupa E, et al. Electrocardiographic abnormalities in patients with acute pulmonary embolism complicated by cardiogenic shock. The American Journal of Emergency Medicine. 2014;**32**(6):507-510

[33] Geibel A, Zehender M, Kasper W, Olschewski M, Klima C, Konstantinides SV. Prognostic value of the ECG on admission in patients with acute major pulmonary embolism. The European Respiratory Journal. 2005;**25**(5):843-848

[34] Kosuge M, Kimura K, Ishikawa T, Ebina T, Hibi K, Kusama I, et al. Electrocardiographic differentiation between acute pulmonary embolism and acute coronary syndromes on the basis of negative T waves. The American Journal of Cardiology. 2007;**99**(6): 817-821

[35] Kosuge M, Ebina T, Hibi K, Tsukahara K, Iwahashi N, Umemura S, et al. Differences in negative T waves between acute pulmonary embolism and acute coronary syndrome. Circulation Journal. 2014;**78**(2):483-489

[36] Kearon C, Ginsberg JS, Hirsh J. The role of venous ultrasonography in the diagnosis of suspected deep venous thrombosis and pulmonary embolism. Annals of Internal Medicine. 1998; **129**(12):1044-1049

[37] Barrellier MT, Lezin B, Landy S, Le Hello C. Prevalence of duplex ultrasonography detectable venous thrombosis in patients with suspected or acute pulmonary embolism. Journal des Maladies Vasculaires. 2001;**26**(1):23-30

[38] Kassai B, Boissel JP, Cucherat M, Sonie S, Shah NR, Leizorovicz A. A systematic review of the accuracy of ultrasound in the diagnosis of deep venous thrombosis in asymptomatic patients. Thrombosis and Haemostasis. 2004;**91**(4):655-666

[39] Strothman G, Blebea J, Fowl RJ, Rosenthal G. Contralateral duplex scanning for deep venous thrombosis is unnecessary in patients with symptoms. Journal of Vascular Surgery. 1995;**22**(5):543-547

[40] Kearon C, Julian JA, Newman TE, Ginsberg JS. Noninvasive diagnosis of deep venous thrombosis. McMaster Diagnostic Imaging Practice Guidelines Initiative. Annals of Internal Medicine. 1998;**128**(8):663-677

[41] Heijboer H, Buller HR, Lensing AW, Turpie AG, Colly LP, Ten Cate JW. A comparison of real-time compression ultrasonography with impedance plethysmography for the diagnosis of deep-vein thrombosis in symptomatic outpatients. The New England Journal of Medicine. 1993;**329**(19):1365-1369

[42] Miniati M, Monti S, Pratali L, Di Ricco G, Marini C, Formichi B, et al. Value of transthoracic echocardiography in the diagnosis of pulmonary embolism: results of a prospective study in unselected patients. The American Journal of Medicine. 2001;**110**(7): 528-535

[43] McConnell MV, Solomon SD, Rayan ME, Come PC, Goldhaber SZ, Lee RT. Regional right ventricular dysfunction detected by echocardiography in acute pulmonary embolism. The American Journal of Cardiology. 1996;**78**(4):469-473

[44] Konstantinides S, Geibel A, Heusel G, Heinrich F, Kasper W, Management S, et al. Heparin plus alteplase compared with heparin alone in patients with submassive pulmonary

embolism. The New England Journal of Medicine. 2002;**347**(15):1143-1150

[45] Grifoni S, Olivotto I, Cecchini P, Pieralli F, Camaiti A, Santoro G, et al. Short-term clinical outcome of patients with acute pulmonary embolism, normal blood pressure, and echocardiographic right ventricular dysfunction. Circulation. 2000;**101**(24):2817-2822

[46] Pruszczyk P, Torbicki A, Kuch-Wocial A, Szulc M, Pacho R. Diagnostic value of transoesophageal echocardiography in suspected haemodynamically significant pulmonary embolism. Heart. 2001;**85**(6):628-634

[47] Fields JM, Davis J, Girson L, Au A, Potts J, Morgan CJ, et al. Transthoracic Echocardiography for Diagnosing Pulmonary Embolism: A Systematic Review and Meta-Analysis. Journal of the American Society of Echocardiography. 2017;**30**(7):714-23 e4

[48] Fesmire FM, Brown MD, Espinosa JA, Shih RD, Silvers SM, Wolf SJ, et al. Critical issues in the evaluation and management of adult patients presenting to the emergency department with suspected pulmonary embolism. Annals of Emergency Medicine. 2011;**57**(6):628-52 e75

[49] Jiang L, Ma Y, Zhao C, Shen W, Feng X, Xu Y, et al. Role of transthoracic lung ultrasonography in the diagnosis of pulmonary embolism: A systematic review and meta-analysis. PLoS One. 2015;**10**(6):e0129909

[50] Comert SS, Caglayan B, Akturk U, Fidan A, Kiral N, Parmaksiz E, et al. The role of thoracic ultrasonography in the diagnosis of pulmonary embolism. Ann Thorac Med. 2013;**8**(2):99-104

[51] Reissig A, Kroegel C. Transthoracic ultrasound of lung and pleura in the diagnosis of pulmonary embolism: a novel non-invasive bedside approach. Respiration. 2003;**70**(5):441-452

[52] Aumiller J, Herth FJ, Krasnik M, Eberhardt R. Endobronchial ultrasound for detecting central pulmonary emboli: A pilot study. Respiration. 2009;**77**(3): 298-302

[53] Stein PD, Henry JW. Prevalence of acute pulmonary embolism among patients in a general hospital and at autopsy. Chest. 1995;**108**(4):978-981

[54] He MC. Dr. Paul Zarogoulidis: The exploration on pneumothorax and new use of EBUS. Journal of Thoracic Disease. 2015;**7**(Suppl 1):S73-S74

[55] Kagima J, Stolbrink M, Masheti S, Mbaiyani C, Munubi A, Joekes E, et al. Diagnostic accuracy of combined thoracic and cardiac sonography for the diagnosis of pulmonary embolism: A systematic review and meta-analysis. PLoS One. 2020;**15**(9):e0235940

[56] Lichtenstein DA, Meziere GA. Relevance of lung ultrasound in the diagnosis of acute respiratory failure: the BLUE protocol. Chest. 2008;**134**(1): 117-125

[57] Koenig S, Chandra S, Alaverdian A, Dibello C, Mayo PH, Narasimhan M. Ultrasound assessment of pulmonary embolism in patients receiving CT pulmonary angiography. Chest. 2014; **145**(4):818-823

[58] Squizzato A, Rancan E, Dentali F, Bonzini M, Guasti L, Steidl L, et al. Diagnostic accuracy of lung ultrasound for pulmonary embolism: A systematic review and meta-analysis. Journal of Thrombosis and Haemostasis. 2013;**11**(7):1269-1278

[59] Ladeiras-Lopes R, Neto A, Costa C, Sousa M, Ferreira P, Dias VP, et al. Hampton's hump and Palla's sign in pulmonary embolism. Circulation. 2013;**127**(18):1914-1915

[60] Abbas A, St Joseph EV, Mansour OM, Peebles CR. Radiographic

features of pulmonary embolism: Westermark and Palla signs. Postgraduate Medical Journal. 2014;**90**(1065):422-423

[61] Lee DS, Vo HA, Franco A, Keshavamurthy J, Rotem E. Palla and Westermark Signs. Journal of Thoracic Imaging. 2017;**32**(4):W7

[62] Investigators P. Value of the ventilation/perfusion scan in acute pulmonary embolism. Results of the prospective investigation of pulmonary embolism diagnosis (PIOPED). JAMA. 1990;**263**(20):2753-2759

[63] Anderson DR, Kahn SR, Rodger MA, Kovacs MJ, Morris T, Hirsch A, et al. Computed tomographic pulmonary angiography vs ventilation-perfusion lung scanning in patients with suspected pulmonary embolism: a randomized controlled trial. JAMA. 2007;**298**(23):2743-2753

[64] Hayashino Y, Goto M, Noguchi Y, Fukui T. Ventilation-perfusion scanning and helical CT in suspected pulmonary embolism: meta-analysis of diagnostic performance. Radiology. 2005;**234**(3): 740-748

[65] Miniati M, Pistolesi M, Marini C, Di Ricco G, Formichi B, Prediletto R, et al. Value of perfusion lung scan in the diagnosis of pulmonary embolism: results of the Prospective Investigative Study of Acute Pulmonary Embolism Diagnosis (PISA-PED). American Journal of Respiratory and Critical Care Medicine. 1996;**154**(5):1387-1393

[66] Henry JW, Stein PD, Gottschalk A, Relyea B, Leeper KV Jr. Scintigraphic lung scans and clinical assessment in critically ill patients with suspected acute pulmonary embolism. Chest. 1996;**109**(2):462-466

[67] van Beek EJ, Brouwers EM, Song B, Bongaerts AH, Oudkerk M. Lung scintigraphy and helical computed tomography for the diagnosis of pulmonary embolism: a meta-analysis. Clinical and Applied Thrombosis/ Hemostasis. 2001;**7**(2):87-92

[68] Hartmann IJ, Hagen PJ, Melissant CF, Postmus PE, Prins MH. Diagnosing acute pulmonary embolism: effect of chronic obstructive pulmonary disease on the performance of D-dimer testing, ventilation/perfusion scintigraphy, spiral computed tomographic angiography, and conventional angiography. ANTELOPE Study Group. Advances in New Technologies Evaluating the Localization of Pulmonary Embolism. American Journal of Respiratory and Critical Care Medicine. 2000;**162**(6): 2232-2237

[69] Revel MP, Cohen S, Sanchez O, Collignon MA, Thiam R, Redheuil A, et al. Pulmonary embolism during pregnancy: Diagnosis with lung scintigraphy or CT angiography? Radiology. 2011;**258**(2):590-598

[70] Roach PJ, Bailey DL, Harris BE. Enhancing lung scintigraphy with single-photon emission computed tomography. Seminars in Nuclear Medicine. 2008;**38**(6):441-449

[71] Harris B, Bailey D, Miles S, Bailey E, Rogers K, Roach P, et al. Objective analysis of tomographic ventilation-perfusion scintigraphy in pulmonary embolism. American Journal of Respiratory and Critical Care Medicine. 2007;**175**(11):1173-1180

[72] Stein PD, Freeman LM, Sostman HD, Goodman LR, Woodard PK, Naidich DP, et al. SPECT in acute pulmonary embolism. Journal of Nuclear Medicine. 2009;**50**(12):1999-2007

[73] Morrell NW, Roberts CM, Jones BE, Nijran KS, Biggs T, Seed WA. The anatomy of radioisotope lung scanning. Journal of Nuclear Medicine. 1992;**33**(5): 676-683

[74] Leblanc M, Leveillee F, Turcotte E. Prospective evaluation of the negative predictive value of V/Q SPECT using 99mTc-Technegas. Nucl Med Commu. 2007;**28**(8):667-672

[75] Roach PJ, Thomas P, Bajc M, Jonson B. Merits of V/Q SPECT scintigraphy compared with CTPA in imaging of pulmonary embolism. Journal of Nuclear Medicine. 2008;**49**(1):167-168 author reply 8

[76] Bajc M, Olsson B, Palmer J, Jonson B. Ventilation/Perfusion SPECT for diagnostics of pulmonary embolism in clinical practice. Journal of Internal Medicine. 2008;**264**(4):379-387

[77] Gutte H, Mortensen J, Jensen CV, Johnbeck CB, von der Recke P, Petersen CL, et al. Detection of pulmonary embolism with combined ventilation-perfusion SPECT and low-dose CT: head-to-head comparison with multidetector CT angiography. Journal of Nuclear Medicine. 2009;**50**(12):1987-1992

[78] Le Roux PY, Robin P, Tromeur C, Davis A, Robert-Ebadi H, Carrier M, et al. Ventilation/perfusion SPECT for the diagnosis of pulmonary embolism: A systematic review. Journal of Thrombosis and Haemostasis. 2020;**18**(11):2910-2920

[79] Hiorns MP, Mayo JR. Spiral computed tomography for acute pulmonary embolism. Canadian Association of Radiologists Journal. 2002;**53**(5):258-268

[80] Reinartz P, Wildberger JE, Schaefer W, Nowak B, Mahnken AH, Buell U. Tomographic imaging in the diagnosis of pulmonary embolism: a comparison between V/Q lung scintigraphy in SPECT technique and multislice spiral CT. Journal of Nuclear Medicine. 2004;**45**(9):1501-1508

[81] Oser RF, Zuckerman DA, Gutierrez FR, Brink JA. Anatomic distribution of pulmonary emboli at pulmonary angiography: implications for cross-sectional imaging. Radiology. 1996;**199**(1):31-35

[82] Stein PD, Henry JW. Prevalence of acute pulmonary embolism in central and subsegmental pulmonary arteries and relation to probability interpretation of ventilation/perfusion lung scans. Chest. 1997;**111**(5):1246-1248

[83] Brenner DJ, Hall EJ. Computed tomography--an increasing source of radiation exposure. The New England Journal of Medicine. 2007;**357**(22): 2277-2284

[84] Hull RD, Raskob GE, Pineo GF, Brant RF. The low-probability lung scan. A need for change in nomenclature. Archives of Internal Medicine. 1995;**155**(17):1845-1851

[85] Stein PD, Chenevert TL, Fowler SE, Goodman LR, Gottschalk A, Hales CA, et al. Gadolinium-enhanced magnetic resonance angiography for pulmonary embolism: A multicenter prospective study (PIOPED III). Annals of Internal Medicine. 2010;**152**(7):434-443 W142-3

[86] Goodman LR, Stein PD, Matta F, Sostman HD, Wakefield TW, Woodard PK, et al. CT venography and compression sonography are diagnostically equivalent: data from PIOPED II. AJR. American Journal of Roentgenology. 2007;**189**(5):1071-1076

[87] Stein PD, Athanasoulis C, Alavi A, Greenspan RH, Hales CA, Saltzman HA, et al. Complications and validity of pulmonary angiography in acute pulmonary embolism. Circulation. 1992;**85**(2):462-468

[88] Wells PS, Anderson DR, Bormanis J, Guy F, Mitchell M, Gray L, et al. Value of assessment of pretest probability of deep-vein thrombosis in clinical management. Lancet. 1997;**350**(9094): 1795-1798

[89] Wells PS, Anderson DR, Rodger M, Forgie M, Kearon C, Dreyer J, et al. Evaluation of D-dimer in the diagnosis of suspected deep-vein thrombosis. The New England Journal of Medicine. 2003;**349**(13):1227-1235

[90] Schutgens RE, Ackermark P, Haas FJ, Nieuwenhuis HK, Peltenburg HG, Pijlman AH, et al. Combination of a normal D-dimer concentration and a non-high pretest clinical probability score is a safe strategy to exclude deep venous thrombosis. Circulation. 2003;**107**(4):593-597

[91] Wicki J, Perneger TV, Junod AF, Bounameaux H, Perrier A. Assessing clinical probability of pulmonary embolism in the emergency ward: a simple score. Archives of Internal Medicine. 2001;**161**(1):92-97

[92] Le Gal G, Righini M, Roy PM, Sanchez O, Aujesky D, Bounameaux H, et al. Prediction of pulmonary embolism in the emergency department: the revised Geneva score. Annals of Internal Medicine. 2006;**144**(3):165-171

[93] Miniati M, Monti S, Bottai M. A structured clinical model for predicting the probability of pulmonary embolism. The American Journal of Medicine. 2003;**114**(3):173-179

[94] Kline JA, Courtney DM, Kabrhel C, Moore CL, Smithline HA, Plewa MC, et al. Prospective multicenter evaluation of the pulmonary embolism rule-out criteria. Journal of Thrombosis and Haemostasis. 2008;**6**(5):772-780

[95] Kline JA, Nelson RD, Jackson RE, Courtney DM. Criteria for the safe use of D-dimer testing in emergency department patients with suspected pulmonary embolism: A multicenter US study. Annals of Emergency Medicine. 2002;**39**(2):144-152

[96] Shen JH, Chen HL, Chen JR, Xing JL, Gu P, Zhu BF. Comparison of the Wells score with the revised Geneva score for assessing suspected pulmonary embolism: A systematic review and meta-analysis. Journal of Thrombosis and Thrombolysis. 2016;**41**(3):482-492

[97] Lax SF, Skok K, Zechner P, Kessler HH, Kaufmann N, Koelblinger C, et al. Pulmonary arterial thrombosis in COVID-19 with fatal outcome : Results from a prospective, single-center, clinicopathologic case series. Annals of Internal Medicine. 2020;**173**(5):350-361

[98] Ackermann M, Verleden SE, Kuehnel M, Haverich A, Welte T, Laenger F, et al. Pulmonary vascular endothelialitis, thrombosis, and angiogenesis in Covid-19. The New England Journal of Medicine. 2020;**383**(2):120-128

[99] Fox SE, Akmatbekov A, Harbert JL, Li G, Quincy Brown J, Vander Heide RS. Pulmonary and cardiac pathology in African American patients with COVID-19: An autopsy series from New Orleans. The Lancet Respiratory Medicine. 2020;**8**(7):681-686

[100] Carsana L, Sonzogni A, Nasr A, Rossi RS, Pellegrinelli A, Zerbi P, et al. Pulmonary post-mortem findings in a series of COVID-19 cases from northern Italy: A two-centre descriptive study. The Lancet Infectious Diseases. 2020;**20**(10):1135-1140

[101] Hariri LP, North CM, Shih AR, Israel RA, Maley JH, Villalba JA, et al. Lung histopathology in coronavirus disease 2019 as compared with severe acute respiratory sydrome and H1N1 influenza: A systematic review. Chest. 2021;**159**(1):73-84

[102] van Dam LF, Kroft LJM, van der Wal LI, Cannegieter SC, Eikenboom J, de Jonge E, et al. Clinical and computed tomography characteristics of COVID-19 associated acute pulmonary embolism: A different phenotype of

thrombotic disease? Thrombosis Research. 2020;**193**:86-89

[103] Girard P, Sanchez O, Leroyer C, Musset D, Meyer G, Stern JB, et al. Deep venous thrombosis in patients with acute pulmonary embolism: Prevalence, risk factors, and clinical significance. Chest. 2005;**128**(3):1593-1600

[104] Lim W, Le Gal G, Bates SM, Righini M, Haramati LB, Lang E, et al. American Society of Hematology 2018 guidelines for management of venous thromboembolism: Diagnosis of venous thromboembolism. Blood Advances. 2018;**2**(22):3226-3256

[105] Wallace A, Albadawi H, Hoang P, Fleck A, Naidu S, Knuttinen G, et al. Statins as a preventative therapy for venous thromboembolism. Cardiovasc Diagn Ther. 2017;7(Suppl 3):S207-SS18

[106] Poyiadji N, Cormier P, Patel PY, Hadied MO, Bhargava P, Khanna K, et al. Acute Pulmonary Embolism and COVID-19. Radiology. 2020;**297**(3): E335-E3E8

[107] Suh YJ, Hong H, Ohana M, Bompard F, Revel MP, Valle C, et al. Pulmonary embolism and deep vein thrombosis in COVID-19: A systematic review and meta-analysis. Radiology. 2021;**298**(2):E70-E80

[108] Helms J, Tacquard C, Severac F, Leonard-Lorant I, Ohana M, Delabranche X, et al. High risk of thrombosis in patients with severe SARS-CoV-2 infection: A multicenter prospective cohort study. Intensive Care Medicine. 2020;**46**(6):1089-1098

[109] Poissy J, Goutay J, Caplan M, Parmentier E, Duburcq T, Lassalle F, et al. Pulmonary embolism in patients With COVID-19: Awareness of an Increased Prevalence. Circulation. 2020;**142**(2):184-186

[110] Zheng KI, Gao F, Wang XB, Sun QF, Pan KH, Wang TY, et al. Letter to the Editor: Obesity as a risk factor for greater severity of COVID-19 in patients with metabolic associated fatty liver disease. Metabolism. 2020;**108**:154244

[111] Di Minno A, Ambrosino P, Calcaterra I, Di Minno MND. COVID-19 and venous thromboembolism: A meta-analysis of literature studies. Seminars in Thrombosis and Hemostasis. 2020;**46**(7):763-771

Chapter 3

Pulmonary Embolism in COVID-19 Patients: Facts and Figures

Nissar Shaikh, Narges Quyyum, Arshad Chanda,
Muhammad Zubair, Muhsen Shaheen, Shajahan Idayatulla,
Sumayya Aboobacker, Jazib Hassan, Shoaib Nawaz,
Ashish Kumar, M.M. Nainthramveetil, Zubair Shahid
and Ibrahim Rasheed

Abstract

COVID-19 infection affects many systems in the body including the coagulation mechanisms. Imbalance between pro-coagulant and anticoagulant activities causes a roughly nine times higher risk for pulmonary embolism (PE) in COVID-19 patients. The reported incidence of PE in COVID-19 patients ranges from 3 to 26%. There is an increased risk of PE in hospitalized patients with lower mobility and patients requiring intensive care therapy. Obesity, atrial fibrillation, raised pro-inflammatory markers, and convalescent plasma therapy increases the risk of PE in COVID-19 patients. Endothelial injury in COVID-19 patients causes loss of vasodilatory, anti-adhesion and fibrinolytic properties. Viral penetration and load leads to the release of cytokines and von Willebrand factor, which induces thrombosis in small and medium vessels. D-dimers elevation gives strong suspicion of PE in COVID-19 patients, and normal D-dimer levels effectively rule it out. Point of care echocardiogram may show right heart dilatation, thrombus in heart or pulmonary arteries. DVT increases the risk of developing PE. The gold standard test for the diagnosis of PE is CTPA (computerized tomographic pulmonary angiography) which also gives alternative diagnosis in the absence of PE. Therapeutic anticoagulation is the corner stone in the management of PE and commonly used anticoagulants are LMWH (low molecular weight heparin) and UFH (unfractionated heparin). Mortality in COVID-19 patients with PE is up to 43% compared to COVID patients without PE being around 3%.

Keywords: COVID-19, computerized tomographic pulmonary angiography, D-dimer, pulmonary embolism, unfractionated heparin, ultrasonography

1. Introduction

COVID-19 infection is primarily a respiratory viral infection, initially described in China and despite restrictive and preventive measures, it spread quickly and within few months became a global pandemic. Although COVID-19 is a respiratory infection, it can cause multiple organ dysfunctions and is thus a constant threat to the life. Hypercoagulable state is a well-known complication particularly in severely ill COVID-19 patients. This increases the risk of thromboembolism, particularly pulmonary embolism (PE) [1]. The presence of pulmonary embolism in COVID-19 patients creates a challenging clinical scenario due to their already compromised respiratory function. Early recognition and therapeutic intervention are critical for better patient management and a positive outcome.

We will discuss the occurrence of PE in COVID-19 infection in following sub-headings.

2. Epidemiology

The incidence of PE in COVID-19 patients is underdiagnosed and varies depending on patient's condition and level of care being provided, but there is an overall 9 folds increased risk of PE in COVID-19 patients compared to the non-COVID population [1]. Overall incidence as well as mortality of PE due to traditional risk factors is decreasing but there are increased incidence and mortality of PE in COVID-19 patients [1]. PE incidence increases further in COVID-19 patients requiring intensive care unit (ICU) admission and one out of three patients in the ICU may have PE. Ng et al. reported the incidence of PE in ICU varies from 3.3 to 26.7% [2]. The evidence of under diagnosis of PE in COVID-19 patients is provided by the fact that a chest CT scan performed in COVID-19 patients regardless of clinical manifestations, showed PE in 50% of the patients [3]. Incidence of PE in COVID-19 patients irrespective of their admission to the hospital or not is reported to be 1.1 to 3.4% [4].

The incidence of PE in the hospitalized patients is reported to be ranging from 1.9 to 8.9% in different studies, being particularly high in critically ill patients (up to 26.6%) [5]. Liu et al. reported that one in five patients with a mean age of 57 years and having comorbid conditions developed PE [6].

3. Risk factors

The risk factors of thromboembolism or PE in COVID-19 patients are not the same as traditional PE risk factors. Traditional risk factors including lower limb fractures, heart failure, hip or knee replacement surgeries, myocardial infarction, spinal trauma, post-partum period do not seem to increase the risk in COVID-19 patients, but sure there will be some relevance of these conditions on the occurrence of PE [7]. African American race and obesity are found to increase the risk of PE in COVID-19 patients. There is no strong relationship between cardiovascular comorbidities and the risk of pulmonary embolism in COVID-19 patients [7]. Various studies reported that the clinical and biological parameters in COVID-19 patients driven by inflammation and coagulopathy increase the risk of PE. Presence of severe inflammation with increase in D-dimers, C-reactive protein (CRP), high fractional inspiration of oxygen and development of ARDS (acute respiratory distress syndrome) were associated with increased risk of PE. Demographic factors increasing risk of PE included male gender, history of stroke, atrial fibrillation, chest pain and dyspnea [7]. COVID-19 patients requiring ECMO (Extracorporeal membrane oxygenation) and convalescent plasma therapy were also at a higher risk of PE [7]. Up to 39% of COVID-19 patients requiring invasive ventilation develop PE [7].

Overall, from the literature it seems that mild to moderate COVID-19 infections, patients with delayed onset of symptoms and hospitalization have increased risk of PE [7, 8].

4. Pathophysiology

COVID-19 and other viral infections generate a hypercoagulable state and thus predispose to thromboembolism. This is caused by activation of systemic inflammatory response syndrome which creates an imbalance between pro and anticoagulant effects. Coagulation and body immune system pathways are essentially interlinked, Thrombin and platelets play an important role in coagulation and immune system stimulation. Blood clot formation limits the loss of immune and blood components, as well as causing slowdown of the microorganisms' invasion of circulation [9]. Endothelial injury in COVID-19 infection leads to loss of vasodilatory, fibrinolysis and anti-aggregation properties. Endothelial injury induced by the local viral load and penetration into the endothelium, releases cytokines and von Willebrand factors, inducing the thrombosis initiation in medium and smaller vessels [9].

Further in the process, release of pro-inflammatory cytokines causes vascular endothelial apoptosis, increases adhesion molecules causing pro-adhesive and proinflamatory effects. Endothelial damage also causes imbalance between ADAMTS-13 (A disintigrin and metalloproteinase with thrombospondin type1 motif memeber13) and excessive generation of ultra large von Willebrand factor multi lumen (ULVWF) from the endothelial cells, the ULVWF adheres to the endothelium surface and recruits platelets causing micro thrombi generation [10].

Secondly the endothelial injury with elevated von Willebrand factor (vWF), toll-like receptor activation and tissue pathway activation induce pro-inflammatory and pro-coagulant state through complement activation and cytokines release resulting in dysregulation of the coagulation process with formation of intra-alveolar and systemic clots [11].

Moreover, the release of higher amount of proinflammatory cytokines causes 'cytokine storm' leading to secondary development of hemophagocytic lympho-histiocytosis and activation of blood clotting with increased risk of micro thrombosis. The final interaction between various blood cells (microphages, monocytes, platelets, lymphocytes, endothelial cells) plays an important role in the pro-coagulant effect in COVID-19 infection. Platelet activation by viral invasion facilitates pathogen clearance by white blood cells and clot formation [12].

5. Diagnosis

The diagnosis of PE in COVID-19 patients is challenging as signs and symptoms of PE are not specific and overlap with COVID-19 respiratory manifestations.

Hence PE is diagnosis is often missed or delayed in COVID-19 patients. As COVID-19 patients may be unstable and have high risk of viral aerosolization, imaging studies may not be practically possible. Initial diagnosis is suspected based upon the physical, clinical and laboratory parameters. If COVID-19 patients have DVT (deep venous thrombosis) patients will have moderate to high chances of developing PE.

Unexplained tachycardia, tachypnea or dyspnea, poor gas exchange or hemodynamic instability and sudden worsening respiratory status should ring an alarm of possible PE diagnosis. Patients with risk factors such as malignancy, on hormonal therapy, having milder x-ray changes, not correlating to or out of proportion to clinical severity of the disease should give high index of suspicion of PE. A study shows that only 33% of COVID-19 patients with PE had a Wells' score of more than 4, hence Wells' score has limited application in COVID-19 patients [13].

ECG (electrocardiography) often shows tachycardia; however, it may reveal right heart strain pattern in severe cases. The point of care echocardiography

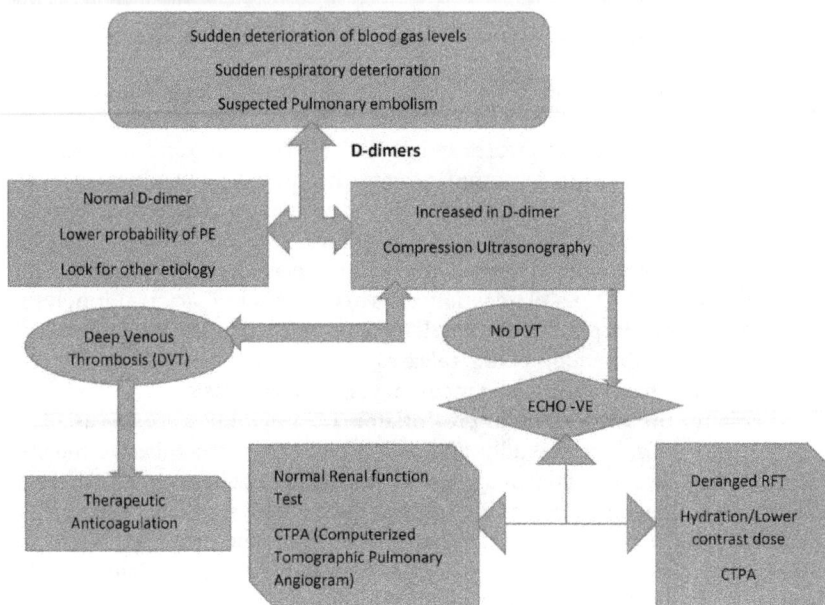

Figure 1.
Diagnostic algorithm for PE in COVID-19 patients.

(POCUS) may show acute right ventricular overload and dilatation, intra-cardiac thrombi, or thrombus transit.

Rapid increase in inflammatory markers and D-dimer levels is commonly associated with the development of PE in COVID-19 patients. Elevated D-dimers were found to be associated with a 50% increased risk of DVT in COVID-19 patients [14]. As these inflammatory markers and D-dimers also elevated in primary or secondary infection, hence recent guidelines advise against using them as association of PE or DVT [15]. Normal D-dimer levels on the contrary are sufficient to rule out DVT or PE with confidence [15].

CTPA (computerized tomographic pulmonary angiography) is specific and sensitive imaging modality to diagnose, confirm or exclude PE. CTPA has an accuracy of 95% in the diagnosis of the PE, and in its absence, gives alternative diagnosis. All infection control precautions, and hemodynamic monitoring should be continued while transporting patients to the imaging suite. **Figure 1** reflects steps wise algorithm for the diagnosis of PE in COVID-19 patients.

6. Management

Therapeutic anticoagulation is the key in the management of PE in COVID-19 patients. Thromboprophylaxis should be started in all patients diagnosed with COVID-19 infection. Selection of anticoagulation medication depends on presence of comorbidities, organ dysfunction or failure. Especial consideration is required in renal, liver, gastrointestinal dysfunction, and thrombocytopenia.

The recommended first line anticoagulants are the LMWH (low molecular weight heparin) due to their obvious benefits, but unfractionated heparin (UFH) is the drug of choice in patients with severe renal impairment, patients expecting surgical intervention or invasive procedures. The reason is that unfractionated heparin has a shorter half-life and is easy to reverse with protamine sulfate. All these patients should have regular monitoring of coagulation parameters and the dose should be titrated accordingly [9].

Direct oral anticoagulants (DOAC) should be avoided in acute phase as the patients' organ dysfunction can potentiate and prolong the DOAC action. Their reversal is not easily available as well. DOAC can be considered in the recovery phase of COVID-19 as they have advantage of not requiring monitoring of coagulation parameters [9].

The use of catheter guided therapies should be limited to the most critical patients in the COVID-19 pandemic [9, 15].

Insertion of inferior vena cava (IVC) filter should be considered in patients with recurrent PE and/or DVT despite optimal anticoagulation or having absolute contraindication for anticoagulation [9]. Thrombolytic therapy is immediate choice if the patient is hemodynamically unstable and/or echocardiogram is showing right heart dilatation or pulmonary hypertension.

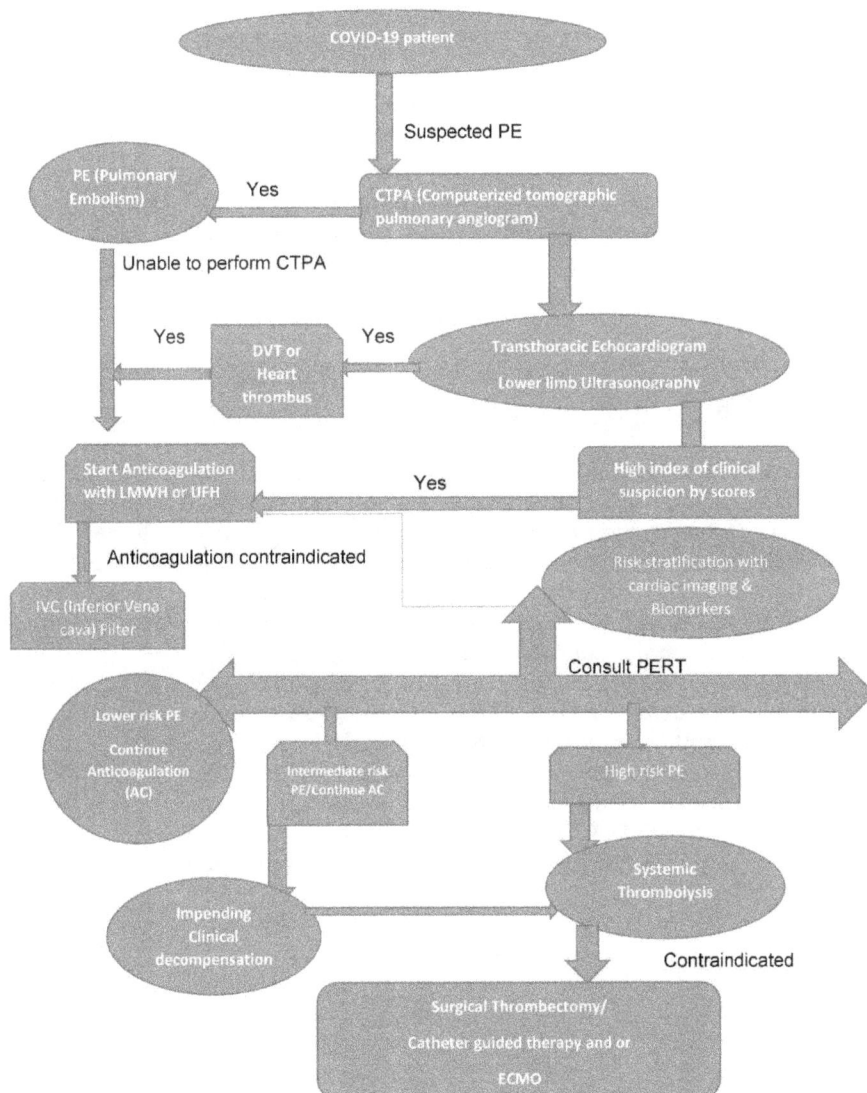

Figure 2.
Management of pulmonary embolism in COVID-19 patients.

In patients with refractory hypoxia or shock or cardiac arrest, ECMO (extracorporeal membrane oxygenation) therapy alone or in combination with thrombectomy or catheter guided thrombolysis is the recommended therapy [9].

All hospitalized COVID-19 patients and patients admitted to ICU should be on thromboprohylaxis, and these patients with increase in inflammatory markers (CRP and Platelets) and D-dimer levels more than 3 ug/ml should be therapeutic dosage of LMWH or UFH depending on their organ dysfunction particularly renal functions [9].

PE managed by PERT (pulmonary embolism response team) may lead to better patient outcomes. PERT not only expedites the diagnosis, but also provides coordinated, multidisciplinary care to PE patients. PERT usually varies in different hospitals and may include an intensivist, cardiothoracic and vascular surgeons, emergency medicine specialist, interventional radiologist, and a clinical pharmacist [16]. PE in COVID-19 patients can be better managed by using an algorithm of care (**Figure 2**).

7. Morbidity and mortality

COVID-19 patients who have PE usually have longer durations of mechanical ventilation, ICU and hospital stay [17]. They have a 45% higher mortality compared to those without PE. Mortality in COVID-19 patients with PE depends on comorbidities, organ dysfunction and length of hospital stay [17]. The mortality is significantly high is first week especially in patients with increased inflammatory markers and may be related to the severity of the disease [17].

8. Conclusion

The risk of PE is quite high in COVID-19 patients. Severe disease requiring hospitalization, ICU admission, obesity, history of atrial fibrillation, cancer and convalescent plasma therapy increases the risk of PE in COVID-19 patients. Endothelial injury in COVID-19 patients occurring due to viral penetration and load causes loss of vasodilatory, anti-adhesive properties and fibrinolysis. It also stimulates the release of cytokines and von Willebrand factor leading to micro thrombi formation in small and medium sized blood vessels.

Diagnosis of PE requires high index of suspicion in COVID-19 patients. Normal D-dimer levels exclude PE with confidence. Bedside transthoracic echocardiography may show right heart dilatation, thrombus in the heart or pulmonary arteries. CTPA is highly sensitive and specific in the diagnosis of PE. If PE is absent CTPA may also give an alternate diagnosis.

Anticoagulation with LMWH and UFH is essential part of the PE management. Few patients may need catheter guided thrombolysis, thrombectomy and/or ECMO therapy.

COVID-19 patients complicated with PE have higher number of days with ventilatory support, ICU and hospital stay. Occurrence of PE in COVID-19 patients also increases the mortality.

Author details

Nissar Shaikh[1*], Narges Quyyum[1], Arshad Chanda[1], Muhammad Zubair[1],
Muhsen Shaheen[2], Shajahan Idayatulla[1], Sumayya Aboobacker[1], Jazib Hassan[1],
Shoaib Nawaz[1], Ashish Kumar[1], M.M. Nainthramveetil[1], Zubair Shahid[3]
and Ibrahim Rasheed[4]

1 Surgical Intensive Care Unit, Hamad Medical Corporation, Doha, Qatar

2 Medical Intensive Care Unit, Hamad Medical Corporation, Doha, Qatar

3 Department of Internal Medicine, Hamad Medical Corporation, Doha, Qatar

4 Pulmonary Medicine, Hamad Medical Corporation, Doha, Qatar

*Address all correspondence to: nissatfirdous99@gmail.com

IntechOpen

References

[1] Òscar Miró, Sònia Jiménez, Alexandre Mebazaa, Yonathan Freund, Guillermo Burillo-Putze, Alfonso Martín, Francisco Javier Martín-Sánchez, Eric Jorge García-Lamberechts, et al. on behalf of the Spanish Investigators on Emergency Situations TeAm (SIESTA) network, Pulmonary embolism in patients with COVID-19: Incidence, risk factors, clinical characteristics, and outcome. European Heart Journal 2021; ehab314.

[2] Ng JJ, Liang ZC, Choong AMTL. The incidence of pulmonary thromboembolism in COVID-19 patients admitted to the intensive care unit: A meta-analysis and meta-regression of observational studies. J Intensive Care. 2021 Feb 22; 9(1):20.

[3] Grillet F, Behr J, Calame P, Aubry S, Delabrousse E. Acute pulmonary embolism associated with COVID-19 pneumonia detected with pulmonary CT angiography. Radiology. 2020; 296(3):E186-E188.

[4] Helms J, Tacquard C, Severac F, Leonard-Lorant I, Ohana M, Delabranche X, et al. CRICS TRIGGERSEP Group (Clinical Research in Intensive Care and Sepsis Trial Group for Global Evaluation and Research in Sepsis). High risk of thrombosis in patients with severe SARS-CoV-2 infection: A multicenter prospective cohort study. Intensive Care Med. 2020; 46(6):1089-1098.

[5] Klok FA, Kruip MJHA, van der Meer NJM, Arbous MS, Gommers D, Kant KM, Kaptein FHJ, van Paassen J, Stals MAM, Huisman MV, Endeman H. Confirmation of the high cumulative incidence of thrombotic complications in critically ill ICU patients with COVID-19: An updated analysis. Thromb Res. 2020; 191:148-150.

[6] Liu K, Fang YY, Deng Y, Liu W, Wang MF, Ma JP, Xiao W, Wang YN, Zhong MH, Li CH, Li GC, Liu HG. Clinical characteristics of novel coronavirus cases in tertiary hospitals in Hubei Province. Chin Med J (Engl). 2020; 133(9):1025-1031.

[7] Akhter MS, Hamali HA, Mobarki AA, Rashid H, Oldenburg J, Biswas A. SARS-CoV-2 infection: Modulator of pulmonary embolism paradigm. J Clin Med. 2021; 10(5):1064.

[8] Martin AI, Rao G. COVID-19: A potential risk factor for acute pulmonary embolism. Methodist Debakey Cardiovasc J. 2020; 16(2):155-157.

[9] Sakr Y, Giovini M, Leone M, Pizzilli G, Kortgen A, Bauer M, Tonetti T, Duclos G, Zieleskiewicz L, Buschbeck S, Ranieri VM, Antonucci E. Pulmonary embolism in patients with coronavirus disease-2019 (COVID-19) pneumonia: A narrative review. Ann Intensive Care. 2020 Sep 16; 10:124.

[10] Varatharajah N, Rajah S. Microthrombotic complications of COVID-19 are likely due to embolism of circulating endothelial derived ultralarge Von Willebrand factor (eULVWF) decorated-platelet strings. Fed Pract. 2020; 37(6):e1-e2.

[11] Matthijs Oudkerk, Harry R. Büller, Dirkjan Kuijpers, Nick van Es, Sytse F. Oudkerk, Theresa McLoud, Diederik Gommers, Jaap van Dissel, Hugo ten Cate, and Edwin J. R. van Beek. Diagnosis, prevention, and treatment of thromboembolic complications in COVID-19: Report of the National Institute for Public Health of the Netherlands. Radiology 2020 297:1, E216-E222.

[12] Giannis D, Ziogas IA, Gianni P. Coagulation disorders in coronavirus infected patients: COVID-19,

SARS-CoV-1, MERS-CoV and lessons
from the past. J Clin Virol. 2020;
127:104362.

[13] Kirsch B, Aziz M, Kumar S, et al.
Wells score to predict pulmonary
embolism in patients with coronavirus
disease 2019. Am J Med. 2021;
134(5):688-690.

[14] Middeldorp S, Coppens M, van
Haaps TF, Foppen M, Vlaar AP,
Müller MCA, Bouman CCS,
Beenen LFM, Kootte RS, Heijmans J,
Smits LP, Bonta PI, van Es N. Incidence
of venous thromboembolism in
hospitalized patients with COVID-19.
J Thromb Haemost. 2020; 18(8):
1995-2002.

[15] Moores LK, Tritschler T,
Brosnahan S, et al. Prevention,
diagnosis, and treatment of VTE in
patients with coronavirus disease 2019:
CHEST guideline and expert panel
report. Chest. 2020; 158(3):1143-1163.

[16] Rosovsky RP, Grodzin C,
Channick R, et al. Diagnosis and
treatment of pulmonary embolism
during the coronavirus disease 2019
pandemic: A position paper from the
National PERT Consortium. Chest.
2020; 158(6):2590-2601.

[17] Bobadilla-Rosado LO, Mier y
Teran-Ellis S, Lopez-Pena G,
Anaya-Ayala JE, Hinojosa CA. Clinical
outcomes of pulmonary embolism in
Mexican patients with COVID-19.
Clinical and Applied Thrombosis/
Hemostasis. 2021; 27:1-4.

Chapter 4

Anticoagulants in the Management of Pulmonary Embolism

Ladan Panahi, George Udeani, Michael Horseman,
Jaye Weston, Nephy Samuel, Merlyn Joseph, Andrea Mora,
Daniela Bazan and Pooja Patel

Abstract

Pulmonary embolism management has typically been accomplished with anticoagulant treatment that includes parenteral heparins and oral vitamin K antagonists. Even though heparins and oral vitamin K antagonists continue to play a role in pulmonary embolism management, other newer available options have somewhat reduced the role of heparins and vitamin K antagonists in pulmonary embolism management. This reduction in utilization involves their toxicity profile, clearance limitations, and many drug and nutrient interactions. New direct oral anticoagulation therapies have led to more available options in the management of pulmonary embolism in the inpatient and outpatient settings. More evidence and research are now available about reversal agents and monitoring parameters regarding these newer agents, leading to more interest in administering them for safe and effective pulmonary embolism management. Current research and literature have also helped direct the selection of appropriate use of pharmacological management of pulmonary embolism based on the specific population such as patients with liver failure, renal failure, malignancy, and COVID-19.

Keywords: pulmonary embolism (PE), venous thromboembolism (VTE), anticoagulants, direct oral anticoagulants (DOAC), heparin, vitamin K antagonist (VKA)

1. Introduction

Pulmonary embolism (PE) is a type of venous thromboembolism (VTE) that is potentially fatal but can be treated with different types of therapy. PE is an obstruction of the pulmonary arteries that can be caused by a clot, tumor, fat, or air. PE occurs when a portion of a blood clot breaks off and travels until it lodges in the pulmonary arteries [1]. Most deep vein thrombosis will develop in the lower extremities, but up to half can lead to PE [2]. PE is a significant health issue in the US, since there is an increased prevalence of this condition in the elderly. Other risk factors include obesity, heart failure, and cancer [3].

Current anticoagulation management guidelines prefer direct oral anticoagulants (DOAC) such as dabigatran, rivaroxaban, apixaban, and edoxaban for initial and long-term therapy for treating PE [4]. DOACs are preferred over vitamin K antagonist (VKA) therapy. This is due to the similar risk reduction for recurrent VTE, reduced risk of bleeding, and improved patient and provider convenience over the intensive monitoring associated with VKA therapy [4]. Each of the DOACs has demonstrated similar efficacy outcomes compared to VKA therapy with recurrent embolism [4]. In contrast, the risk of bleeding differs with the DOACs, which demonstrate less risk when compared to warfarin [4]. One possible exception to this, however, is that gastrointestinal bleeding may be higher with dabigatran, rivaroxaban, and edoxaban compared to warfarin. This has been observed in patients treated with atrial fibrillation [4]. Treatment recommendations differ when managing PE in special populations such as cancer, pregnancy, obesity, elderly, renal dysfunction, hepatic dysfunction, and COVID-19. Low-molecular-weight heparin (LMWH) is recommended over VKA therapy in cancer-associated thrombosis. Evidence suggests that LMWH is more effective in reducing recurrent embolism in this population and is more reliable in patients who have difficulty tolerating oral intake. It further removed the need for frequent monitoring of the international normalized ratio (INR) [4]. The prevention of PE in hospitalized patients includes either LMWH, low-dose unfractionated heparin (UFH) administered twice or three times daily, or fondaparinux [5]. Bleeding remains a concern with anticoagulation therapy. With the availability of reversal agents, clinicians have been able to push the boundaries of PE management with confidence in both the inpatient and outpatient settings.

The duration of anticoagulant therapy for PE is 3 months, at minimum, which may be extended or indefinite in selected circumstances [4]. In patients with a PE provoked by surgery or a nonsurgical transient risk factor, the recommended duration of anticoagulation is 3 months [4]. In patients with an unprovoked PE, bleeding risk determines the duration, but in patients with high bleeding risk, the duration remains at 3 months. In low to moderate bleeding risk, the duration of therapy becomes indefinite [4].

2. Unfractionated heparin (UFH)

UFH is a parenteral anticoagulant that works by inactivating thrombin (IIa) and factor Xa *via* antithrombin. It is derived from porcine or bovine tissue. UFH is the anticoagulant of choice in patients with PE who have a high bleeding risk, critical illness, or need a surgical/invasive procedure. This is due to its short half-life that ranges from 0.5 to 1.5 h, leading to the anticoagulant effect's rapid onset and offset within hours of IV discontinuation [6]. Furthermore, due to its unique metabolism and clearance through the reticuloendothelial system, it is a desirable option for patients with poor and/or unstable renal function (creatinine clearance (CrCL) < 30 mL/min) [1]. Lastly, UFH lacks cytochrome P450 enzyme activity in the liver, and hence, drug interactions are predominantly limited to increased bleeding risk with concurrent anticoagulant and antiplatelet therapy. This makes it a favorable agent in patients with concerns of drug–drug interactions [7].

The IV route is the preferred mode of administration in shock and/or hypotension due to the absorption variability from subcutaneous tissues secondary to UFH plasma protein binding [6]. Dosing and special considerations for UFH are discussed in **Table 1**.

Some adverse drug reactions of concern are thrombocytopenia and major bleeding, such as intracranial and gastrointestinal bleeds. Heparin-associated thrombocytopenia can present in two forms. There is an early, benign, reversible nonimmune thrombocytopenia form and a late, more serious immunoglobulin G

Drug	Dose	Special considerations
UFH [1]	80 unit/kg IV bolus, followed by an 18-unit/kg/h infusion [6].	
Enoxaparin	1 mg/kg subQ [2] BID [3] [8, 9].	
Dalteparin	200 IU/kg/day [4] subQ for one month, followed by 150 IU/kg/day subcutaneously for months 2 through 6 [10].	Maximum of 18,000 IU per day.
Fondaparinux	<50 kg:5 mg subQ daily 50–100 mg: 7.5 mg subQ daily >100 kg: 10 mg subQ daily	Initiate warfarin within 72 h and give concomitantly for at least 5 days.
Edoxaban	60 mg po once daily; 30 mg once daily if body weight ≤ 60 kg	Not for use in patients with CrCl >95 mL/min [5]. Dose after 5 to 10 days of initial therapy with a parenteral anticoagulant.
Apixaban	10 mg po twice daily for 7 days followed by 5 mg twice daily [11].	
Rivaroxaban	15 mg po twice daily x 3 weeks, then 20 mg once daily x at least 6 months [12].	Take with food to improve absorption [13–15]
Dabigatran	150 mg po BID [16].; 110 mg BID for patients ≥80 years	Dose after 5 to 10 days of initial therapy with a parenteral anticoagulant. Reduce dose to 110 mg BID for patients ≥80 years or ≥ 75 years with at least one bleeding risk factor.

[1]UFH: unfractionated heparin.
[2]subQ: subcutaneously.
[3]BID: twice a day.
[4]IU: international units.
[5]CrCL: creatinine clearance.

Table 1.
Anticoagulant dosing and special considerations.

(IgG)-mediated immune thrombocytopenia type, referred to as heparin-induced thrombocytopenia (HIT). HIT poses a concern with UFH use in the treatment of PE, with the overall incidence being reported to be up to 7% in patients with a mortality of 20–30% and varies depending on factors such as patient population (surgical vs. medicine), duration of heparin use, and the type of heparin administered [17, 18]. UFH has a threefold higher risk of HIT compared to LMWH and serious limb-threatening and life-threatening complications [19]. The mechanism of HIT stems from IgG formation against the heparin/PF4 complex on platelets. Once IgG binds to the heparin/PF4 complex on platelets, the platelets become activated, resulting in venous and arterial thrombi formation [19, 20]. Monitoring platelets every 2–4 days or more frequently in higher-risk patients is recommended in patients on treatment doses of heparin [20]. Another side effect of concern is the significant reduction in bone density reported in about 30% of adult patients and the symptomatic bone fractures that occur in 2–3% of adult patients receiving heparin for at least 1 month or more [21].

A complete outline of first line and alternate reversal agents utilized for anticoagulants for PE management is outlined in **Table 2**. Protamine sulfate is a reversal agent indicated for the reversal of UFH- and LMWH-associated bleeds. This agent is administered by a slow IV infusion at doses <5 mg/min due to the concerns of anaphylaxis, hypotension, bradycardia, and respiratory toxicity associated with the rapid infusion [8]. Due to UFH's short half-life, a reversal agent may not be necessary for most cases, as the UFH effect will normalize due to its rapid clearance [8].

	First-line reversal agent	Alternative reversal agents
UFH [1]	Protamine sulfate	
LMWH [2]	Protamine sulfate	
VKA [3]	4F-PCC [4]	FFP [5]
Dabigatran	Idarucizumab	PCC [6]
		aPCC [7]
Direct oral factor-Xa inhibitors	Andexanet alfa	PCC
		aPCC
Fondaparinux	Factor VIIa	aPCC
		Andexanet alfa

[1]UFH: Unfractionated heparin.
[2]LMWH: low molecular weight heparin.
[3]VKA: vitamin K antagonist.
[4]4F-PCC: 4-factor prothrombin complex concentrate.
[5]FFP: fresh-frozen plasma.
[6]PCC: prothrombin complex concentrate.
[7]aPCC: activated prothrombin complex concentrate.

Table 2.
Recommended reversal agents for anticoagulant therapy.

3. Low-molecular-weight heparins (LMWH)

LMWHs, including enoxaparin and dalteparin, are defined as having a mean molecular weight that is less than 50% of that of UFH. They offer the advantage of consistent anticoagulant effect administered subcutaneously and dosing by body weight. Dosing and special considerations for LMWH (enoxaparin and dalteparin) are discussed in **Table 1**. LMWH is currently the preferred anticoagulant for active malignancy and pregnancy. However, newer study findings support the notion that DOACs may benefit VTE treatment in cancer patients [9].

Thrombocytopenia and major bleeding are also possible adverse effects of concern. While the risk of HIT is lower with LMWH in comparison with UFH, a baseline platelet count is suggested as a basis from which to contemplate the development of HIT. Further treatment with LMWH should be avoided in patients with a known history of HIT. Although it less likely to trigger the formation of HIT antibodies than UFH, LMWHs are just as effective as UFH in triggering platelet activation by HIT antibodies [21].

Routine anti-Xa monitoring is generally not recommended for enoxaparin but can be considered in patients with severe or unstable renal function and obese patients with a BMI $\geq$ 40 kg/m^2 (or > 190 kg) who will be on enoxaparin for longer than 1 to 2 weeks [8, 9]. The anti-Xa level peak is drawn 4 h after the enoxaparin dose is administered when a steady state is achieved with a target range of 0.6–1.0 IU/mL [9, 22]. Monitoring anti-Xa activity in morbidly obese patients >120–140 kg and patients with severe or unstable renal function may be considered for dalteparin with a target anti-Xa range of 0.5–1.5 IU/mL [10]. Similar to enoxaparin, the anti-Xa levels in patients taking dalteparin must be drawn 4–6 h after the dalteparin dose is administered and once a steady state is achieved (receiving at least 3 to 4 doses) [10].

LMWHs are only partially reversed by protamine (60 to 80%), since binding only occurs with long, large-molecular-weight heparin proteins [8]. Due to its small size, fondaparinux is not reversed by protamine [8]. Protamine is known to interact with platelets, fibrinogen, and other plasma proteins. This may result in an anticoagulant effect of its own; thus, the minimal amount of protamine required to neutralize heparin present in the plasma should be administered [8].

4. Vitamin K antagonist (VKA)

VKA such as warfarin is a vitamin K receptor antagonist that continues to play a role in PE treatment, particularly in patients with severe renal insufficiency, antiphospholipid syndrome, and financial constraints who are unable to afford DOACs [23]. International normalized ratio (INR) monitoring is recommended for warfarin monitoring [24]. Due to the drug's long half-life, slow depletion of factor II, and rapid depletion of anticoagulant protein C, patients are bridged with UFH, LMWH, or fondaparinux for at least 5 days and until the INR reaches the therapeutic range of 2 to 3 [25].

Frequent monitoring may be a barrier to initiating this agent. Furthermore, several food and drug interactions may also limit the desire to initiate warfarin for long-term therapy. Food that is high in vitamin K content such as oils, fats, liver, nuts, and green vegetables may decrease the efficacy of warfarin. Medications that are inducers and inhibitors of CYP2C9, 2C19, 1A2, and 3A4 must require dose adjustments and/or more frequent monitoring of their INR. For these reasons, patients are educated about maintaining consistency with their vitamin K intake and encouraged to discuss any dietary or medication changes with their healthcare provider [26].

Vitamin K is recommended for warfarin reversal if the INR is >10 without significant bleeding and with repeated vitamin K doses every 6–24 h as needed [27]. Vitamin K can be administered by IV or the oral route, with a preference for oral administration; there is an associated risk of anaphylactoid reactions in 3 out of 10,000 patients when IV formulations were administered [28]. Subcutaneous injection is not recommended due to a delayed and unpredictable effect [27]. The availability of 4F-PCC (KCentra®) during the last decade has resulted in its use over FFP as a reversal agent for warfarin-associated bleeding complications. This agent has been employed especially for life-threatening bleeding, where 4F-PCC has demonstrated 25 times more potency in replacing vitamin K-dependent clotting factors than FFP [29]. The limitations of FFP in comparison with 4F-PCC include its slower onset, risks of allergic reaction and infection transmission, blood group compatibility, longer preparation time, and higher volume [29]. A major advantage of 4F-PCCs is their ability to be stored at room temperature as a lyophilized powder and the fact that they can quickly be reconstituted and administered [29]. With life-threatening bleeding, the addition of vitamin K 5 to 10 mg by slow IV infusion is suggested [30].

5. Factor Xa inhibitor injectable

Fondaparinux (Arixtra®) is a synthetic pentasaccharide anticoagulant selectively inhibiting factor Xa *via* antithrombin-dependent actions with no inhibition of thrombin (factor IIa) [31]. Unlike LMWH and UFH, fondaparinux inhibits a targeted step in the coagulation cascade that leads to its anticoagulant effect [31]. Fondaparinux is currently approved in the United States for the treatment of PE in conjunction with warfarin [31]. Dosing and special considerations for fondaparinux are discussed in **Table 1**.

The most common adverse reaction associated with the use of fondaparinux is bleeding complications. While most other agents used for PE management do have a reversal agent, this medication does not. Fondaparinux does not require laboratory monitoring. However, periodic complete blood count, serum creatinine level, stool occult tests, and anti-Xa level can be monitored on an individual basis [31].

For fondaparinux, recombinant activated factor VII and aPCC have some data in human and animal studies, respectively, as reversal agents. Both andexanet alfa (a recombinant factor Xa) and aripazine have been shown to bind to Xa inhibitors but lack any human data with fondaparinux [32].

6. Direct oral anticoagulant (DOACs)

6.1 Apixaban

Apixaban is an oral direct factor Xa inhibitor approved for the treatment and prevention of DVT and PE [11]. Dosing and special considerations for apixaban use for PE treatment are discussed in **Table 1**. The oral bioavailability is approximately 50%, with most of the drug absorption occurring in the small intestine [33]. Drug elimination occurring *via* the metabolism through the CYP3A4 systems in the intestine and liver and the P-glycoprotein system can be enhanced through drug–drug interactions [23, 26, 31, 33–35]. Once absorbed, the terminal half-life ranges between 8 and 12 h, with a steady state achieved within 3 days [23, 26, 31, 33–35]. The premature discontinuation of any anticoagulant, including apixaban, increases the risk of thrombotic events and is listed as a black box warning [11]. Epidural or spinal hematomas may occur in patients treated with apixaban in neuraxial anesthesia or spinal puncture. These hematomas have long-term consequences, such as permanent paralysis. Such risks should be taken into account when patients on apixaban therapy are scheduled for spinal procedures [11].

Andexanet alfa (Andexxa®) can be used to reverse apixaban (off-label) in life-threatening or uncontrollable bleeding. The dosing is based on the specific factor Xa agent-inhibitor to be reversed, dose, and the time since the last dose was administered [36]. Andexanet alfa 400 mg intravenous bolus is administered at a rate of 30 mg/min, followed by 4 mg/min *via* continuous infusion for up to 120 min, to reverse apixaban (5 mg or less) or rivaroxaban (10 mg or less), administered within 8 h or if the time is unknown [36]. High-dose andexanet alfa is also indicated for apixaban doses of greater than 5 mg, or, if unknown, administered within 8 h or an unknown time. The high-dose andexanet alfa regimen is 800 mg intravenous bolus at a target rate of 30 mg/min, followed by 8 mg/min continuous infusion for up to 120 min [36]. The safety and efficacy of administering more than one dose of any of these regimens have not been established [36]. In the absence of either idarucizumab or andexanet alfa for DOAC reversal, administering prothrombin complex concentrate (PCC) or activated prothrombin complex concentrate (aPCC) is alternative to consider. This is based on the limited available human and animal *in vitro* studies [29]. Activated charcoal for the known recent ingestion of DOACs may also be effective when DOAC ingestion occurs within the last 2–4 h [29].

6.2 Rivaroxaban

Rivaroxaban is an oral direct factor Xa inhibitor approved for the prevention and treatment of DVT and PE. Dosing and special considerations for rivaroxaban use for PE treatment are discussed in **Table 1**. The oral bioavailability ranges from approximately 80 to 100% for a 10 mg dose and up to 66% for a 20 mg [37–39]. Bioavailability of doses ≥15 mg is improved with food [37–39]. Renal elimination accounts for approximately 36% of unchanged drug, its use in patients with a

CrCL <30 mL/min is not advised, and <15 mL/min employment is contraindicated [37–39]. Rivaroxaban is not dialyzable [37–39]. Rivaroxaban follows a similar elimination pattern to that of apixaban, with metabolism through the CYP3A4 systems accounting for 57% elimination [37–39]. P-glycoprotein system inhibitors may lead to elevated rivaroxaban serum levels [33, 35, 40]. Rivaroxaban's terminal half-life ranges between 5 and 9 h, with a prolonged half-life of 11–13 h seen in elderly patients [37–39]. The steady-state concentrations for this agent tend to occur within 3 days. The premature discontinuation of any anticoagulant, including rivaroxaban, increases the risk of thrombotic events and is listed as a black box warning [12]. To minimize this risk, an alternate coverage should be considered, should rivaroxaban be discontinued for a reason apart from pathological bleeding or therapy completion [12]. Epidural or spinal hematomas have been observed in patients managed with rivaroxaban undergoing neuraxial anesthesia or spinal puncture. Such hematomas are known to result in long-term or permanent paralysis [12].

Andexanet alfa (Andexxa®) can also be used to reverse rivaroxaban (off-label) in life-threatening or uncontrollable bleeding. Rivaroxaban doses of greater than 10 mg, or if an unknown amount is administered within 8 h or at an unknown time, are managed with the high-dose andexanet alfa regimen [36].

6.3 Dabigatran

Dabigatran (Pradaxa®) is a direct thrombin (IIa) inhibitor approved for the prevention and treatment of DVT and PE. Dosing and special considerations for dabigatran use for PE treatment are discussed in **Table 1**. Dabigatran should be initiated 0–2 h before the next dose of parenteral anticoagulant would have been due, or at the time of discontinuation of UFH continuous infusion [16]. The medication has low oral bioavailability and undergoes hepatic metabolism. P-glycoprotein (P-gp) inducers, such as phenobarbital, rifampin, and fosphenytoin, reduce exposure to dabigatran and should be avoided [16]. In contrast, P-glycoprotein (P-gp) inhibitors increase exposure to dabigatran, and recommendations vary based on the P-gp inhibitor and the indication for dabigatran use [16]. Renal impairment and P-gp inhibition are the major independent risk factors for increased dabigatran exposure and increased risk of bleeding. Hence, renal function assessment at baseline and periodically thereafter is recommended. Dose adjustments for dabigatran doses in patients with severe renal impairment (CrCl 30 mL/min or less) are recommended. Caution must be used in the elderly, as the risk of stroke and bleeding increases with age, as seen in an analysis of the RE-LY (Randomized Evaluation of Long-Term Anticoagulant Therapy) trial [41]. Dabigatran is contraindicated for use in patients with mechanical heart valves. The RE-ALIGN (Randomized, Phase II Study to Evaluate the sAfety and Pharmacokinetics of oraL dabIGatran Etexilate in Patients after Heart Valve replacement) trial was terminated early due to thromboembolic events (valve thrombosis, stroke, and myocardial infarction), and major bleeding was observed in the dabigatran group compared to the warfarin group in heart valve patients [42].

Besides major and minor bleeding, gastrointestinal adverse effects have been reported in studies at an incidence rate ranging from 24.7 to 35% [16]. The gastrointestinal adverse effects reported include but are not limited to dyspepsia, gastritis, abdominal pain or discomfort, and epigastric discomfort [16]. Due to the prevalence of these adverse effects, it is necessary to educate the patient about the potential side effects and advise them not to abruptly discontinue the medication before notifying their healthcare provider [16].

One distinguishing feature of dabigatran is the increase in bioavailability by 75% that occurs if the capsule is broken, chewed, or emptied out of the capsule shell [16].

This leads to an increased risk of toxicity, such as major bleeds [16]. Since the capsule cannot be manipulated due to the stated reason, the medication should not be administered *via* a feeding tube of any type [16]. The medication must be kept in its original container. It must be discarded after 4 months from the date the package was opened due to the lack of stability with light or humidity exposure that may lead to product breakdown and potency loss [16].

There is a specific reversal agent approved for dabigatran. The agent named idarucizumab (Praxbind®) is a monoclonal antibody with 350 times more affinity for dabigatran than thrombin [10, 43]. Diuresis may also help with the excretion of dabigatran as well [16].

6.4 Edoxaban

Edoxaban is an oral direct factor-X inhibitor approved in the United States for the treatment of PE. Approval was based primarily on the Hokusai VTE study, which evaluated 3319 patients with PE. The trial showed that edoxaban was not inferior to warfarin but had a lower bleeding risk [44]. Dosing and special considerations for edoxaban use for PE treatment are discussed in **Table 1**. The oral bioavailability is approximately 60%, and renal elimination accounts for approximately 50% of unchanged drug. Edoxaban's terminal half-life ranges between 10 and 14 h. Interestingly, edoxaban blood levels are lower in patients with better renal function averaging about 40% less in patients with CrCL >95 mL/min when compared to those with CrCl >50 to ≤80 mL/min [45]. Bleeding complications such as hemorrhage (major or minor) appear to be the most common adverse effects associated with edoxaban use [45, 46]. Lastly, andexanet alfa (Andexxa®) can also be used to reverse edoxaban (off-label) in life-threatening or uncontrollable bleeding [36].

7. Thrombolytic therapy

Thrombolytic therapy for PE may be administered systemically or directed by a catheter into the pulmonary arteries to accelerate the resolution of acute PE. Thrombolytic therapy can lower pulmonary artery pressure and increase arterial oxygenation [23]. Studies limiting thrombotic therapy in acute PE have shown the best outcomes by restricting it to patients presenting with a massive (high-risk) PE [23, 47]. Patients presenting with hemodynamic instability, right ventricular dysfunction, and without significant risk of bleeding are considered potential candidates for emergency thrombolytic therapy [4, 48]. The results from timely administration of thrombolytic therapy may be seen within 36 h [49]. Mortality rates occur in up to 30% of patients categorized as high risk and make the timing of therapeutic intervention critical [50–52]. Adverse events, especially the high incidence of bleeding and hemorrhagic stroke, require careful consideration prior to starting thrombolytic therapy [53, 54]. Systemic alteplase (Activase®) is the only FDA-approved thrombolytic for the management of acute massive (high risk) hemodynamically unstable PE [55]. All anticoagulants must be stopped prior to the initiation of alteplase and 100 mg IV infused over 2 h is the most common regimen. Alternative weight-based regimens for patients weighing <65 kg may be considered [56]. A weight-based regimen with a 15 mg bolus followed by 0.75 mg/kg over 30 min (max 50 mg) and then 0.5 mg/kg over the next 30 min (max 35 mg) have shown efficacy without increased bleeding [56]. Intra-catheter-directed alteplase 0.5–2 mg/h for 2–15 h for a total dose of 4–24 mg has been used successfully in facilities by experienced physicians and well-designed protocols, but this route of administration is not FDA approved [57]. Tenecteplase (TNKase®) and reteplase

(Retavase®) have been used for acute massive (high risk) PE, but are not FDA approved for use in patients with PE [58, 59].

8. Monitoring parameters for anticoagulation therapy

Therapeutic anticoagulation is the gold standard for the management of VTE. The narrow therapeutic efficacy window creates challenges in drug selection and monitoring to deliver the appropriate dose to prevent further embolic events while not causing a life-threatening bleed. Historically, guidelines in VTE management include the option of continuous UFH; however, LMWH and direct factor Xa inhibitors have begun to displace UFH as first-line agents [1, 5, 16]. Traditionally, aPTT has served as the marker of therapeutic anticoagulation in patients with VTE due to the exclusive use of UFH [60–67]. Despite decades of experience with aPTT values, challenges in the precision monitoring of anticoagulation continue to create therapeutic dilemmas for clinicians [61, 62]. The lack of standardized methods in monitoring and individualized patient factors, including biological variables and heparin resistance, are credited as most problematic when using aPTT to measure the effect of UFH [63, 64]. While aPTT values remain the standard for measuring the effects of UFH, anti-factor Xa (anti-Xa) heparin assay (HA) is recommended as a monitoring option in place of aPTT values by the American College of Chest Physicians (ACCP) and the College of American Pathologists (CAP) [16, 46]. Anti-Xa levels demonstrate greater consistency in measuring anticoagulation, since they are based on the functional activity of all heparins [66, 67]. Comparatively, the aPTT test measures the function of the intrinsic and common pathways of the coagulation cascade, which can have significant variability among individuals [45, 62, 63].

The implementation of heparin dosing protocols has improved the uniformity of therapeutic anticoagulation with UFH. Most of these protocols are "weight-based," and changes in the units of UFH per hour are adjusted based on the aPTT values [68]. This method of dosing UFH has led to concerns regarding both "over" and "under" anticoagulation using aPTT-level directed therapy. Combining aPTT and anti-Xa levels has been proposed as a method to overcome the variable swings commonly seen in patients with multiple comorbidities, obesity, older age (>70 years), 16 drug-induced coagulopathies, pharmacokinetic changes, and preexisting genetic alterations [44, 45, 60, 62, 65–67]. Some hospital systems have transitioned from the use of aPTT to anti-Xa HA altogether and are reporting the faster attainment of therapeutic anticoagulation in addition to the elimination of multiple laboratory tests and dosage changes [66].

Based on numerous studies, anti-Xa levels have been shown to be a viable alternative to aPTT to achieve and maintain therapeutic anticoagulant levels with UFH [42, 60, 63, 68–70]. Anti-Xa levels have provided a more consistent method of monitoring a patient's response to UFH and demonstrate fewer blood samples and dosage adjustments compared to aPTT values [62, 67].

INR monitoring is recommended more frequently upon warfarin initiation (once a day) and can be extended to typically once a month once INR is stable and in a therapeutic range [26].

Routine laboratory monitoring is not indicated for DOAC, but anti-factor Xa (FXa) can be useful for excluding clinically important levels of DOAC [29]. Edoxaban may elevate the PT and aPTT, but FXa activity may be a better measure of effectiveness [46]. Fondaparinux does not require laboratory monitoring as well. Anti-factor Xa activity is probably the assay for monitoring fondaparinux but is not usually obtained in real time [32]. For the qualitative assessment of dabigatran, thrombin time (TT) and aPTT may be used, with TT being sensitive to dabigatran even at low drug concentrations [29].

9. Special population

9.1 Obesity

Anticoagulant dosing of obese patients with PE remains to be an area that has not been well studied [71]. The bulk of the data comes from pharmacokinetic/pharmacodynamic (PK/PD) studies and subgroup analyses of premarketing trials comparing obese patients to patients with normal body weight [29, 32, 71, 72]. Furthermore, warfarin appears to have the most robust data available in this population. Warfarin pharmacokinetics have been compared in various studies of obese patients with a BMI > 30 and 40 kg/m^2 to normal body weight subjects. These studies found that obesity was associated with a greater delay and dosage to achieve a therapeutic INR. Data associated with the risk of bleeding, however, have been conflicting, indicating that obesity may or may not increase the risk [71]. While warfarin has the most robust data in this population, the usage of warfarin appears to be on the decline [71].

Dabigatran is a direct thrombin inhibitor that sets it apart from other DOACs. Subgroup analyses of Phase 3 trials for VTE (RE-LY) and atrial fibrillation (RECOVER) suggested no significant differences in the efficacy and safety outcomes of obese patients in comparison with those with lower body weights [29, 32]. In contrast, treatment failures have been documented in morbidly obese patients using standard doses. The authors reported that standard doses failed to achieve "therapeutic levels," suggesting a higher volume of distribution (Vd) and a higher clearance [27, 28].

The factor X inhibitors, rivaroxaban, apixaban, and edoxaban also have some data in obese populations. Rivaroxaban was evaluated in a small PK/PD study involving a heterogeneous group of subjects including those in the obese range (>120 kg). The half-life, Vd, and clearance declined slightly with increasing body weight. The authors felt the declines were not clinically relevant [30]. A separate PK/PD analysis using pooled data from the phase ll EINSTEIN DVT and ODIXa-DVT trials reported similar findings. These studies enrolled some patients with BMIs >35 kg/m^2 and found clinical benefits comparable across all weight groups [36]. The authors of this analysis also concluded that standard doses should be sufficient to treat obese patients; however, a review questioned whether the data were robust enough to draw that conclusion [36, 72].

In the apixaban's phase 1 PK/PD study, the pharmacokinetic data were somewhat different compared to those for rivaroxaban. The overall Vd was higher in subjects >120 kg or BMI > 30 kg/m^2 than normal body weight subjects. The half-life declined almost proportionately to the increase in Vd (27% ↓ vs. 24% ↑ for half-life and Vd, respectively). Peak level and area under the plasma drug concentration-time curve (AUC) were also reduced in the higher body weight subjects. The authors concluded the differences were unlikely to be of clinical significance [47]. The phase 3 trials, ARISTOTLE and AMPLIFY, contained a significant proportion of patients with body weights >100 kg and BMIs above 30 kg/m^2. Subgroup analyses found no differences in efficacy; however, more bleeding episodes were reported in the ARISTOTLE trial. Whether the increase in hemorrhagic complications between these trials was due to age, renal clearance, or other patient-specific factors is unclear [48–50].

Edoxaban has less data than other DOACs. Phase 3 Hokusai-VTE enrolled a large group of patients >100 kg. There was no difference in efficacy and safety compared to groups with other weights [51].

A recent international retrospective study of LMWHs examined dosing in obesity regarding capped (<18,000 IU/d) and uncapped dosages (>18,000 IU/d). The data were obtained from the RIETE Registry, a large prospective case series of patients with VTE. LMWHs included enoxaparin, dalteparin, and tinzaparin. The authors reported that the results may be subject to selection bias despite attempts to control for potential confounders in multivariable analysis. Nevertheless, they found that after adjustment for multiple potential confounders, patients with obesity (>100 kg or BMI >30 kg/m^2) who received capped doses were at a lower risk of having the composite outcome of VTE recurrences, major bleeding, or all-cause death at 15 and 90 days. Bleeding was also reduced with capped dosages [52].

A recent retrospective study of UFH for acute venous thromboembolism (VTE) compared three body mass index (BMI) cohorts: (i) non-obese (less than 30 kg/m^2), (ii) obese (30 to 39.9 kg/m^2), and (iii) morbid obesity ($\geq$40 kg/m^2). The dosing employed was based on actual body weight. The median times to therapeutic aPTT were reported as 16.4, 16.6, and 17.1 h in each of the three cohorts [53].

Obese patients on warfarin may require a higher dose or more time to achieve a therapeutic INR. Bleeding risk may or may not be greater. Available data for DOACs other than dabigatran suggested usual doses may not negatively impact efficacy in obese patients. Apixaban studies reported conflicting results on bleeding risk. However, there are probably insufficient data for DOACs to suggest that usual doses would be adequate in the subgroup of morbidly obese patients. Obese patients with capped doses of LMWHs may have better efficacy and safety outcomes. Capped dosages are conditionally recommended in the 2018 American Society of Hematology guidelines [54].

9.2 Renal dysfunction

Anticoagulants have been evaluated in CKD and ESKD patients in various PK/PD and clinical efficacy trials [55]. The PK/PD of warfarin in CKD and ESKD is not completely understood [55, 56]. Official dosing guidelines do not recommend an alteration of dose [55]. Warfarin is extensively metabolized by the cytochrome P450 type 2C9 (CYP2C9) enzyme [73]. Although not removed by dialysis, there are no data evaluating whether this procedure alters its pharmacokinetics and pharmacodynamics [55]. One study comparing individuals with a GFR of 30–59 mL/min and healthy controls reported a shorter half-life and increased clearance. Other data showed that CKD, especially GFRs <30 mL/min per 1.73 m^2 or ESKD, complicates warfarin therapy [58, 59]. These data reported that lower doses were required to maintain therapeutic INR with greater fluctuations in INR values and higher risks of major bleeding events for any given INR value. A recent meta-analysis of ESKD patients with atrial fibrillation found that warfarin had no benefit in reducing ischemic stroke incidence. The authors concluded that the drug appeared to be associated with a significantly higher risk of hemorrhagic stroke but no increased risk of other types of major bleeding. They also found no change in mortality [71, 74]. How all these data apply to other indications such as PE is unknown.

The various DOACS have also been evaluated in renal disease. A small study of dabigatran using reduced doses (150 mg daily for CKD and 50 mg daily for ESKD) examined the effect of CKD and ESKD on pharmacokinetic parameters. Subjects with a creatinine clearance <30 mL/min demonstrated a 6.5-time increase in the AUC with a doubling of the half-life compared to normal controls [75].

Rivaroxaban has somewhat conflicting data in CKD and ESKD. In a phase 3 trial subgroup analysis of the Rivaroxaban Once Daily Oral Direct Factor Xa Inhibition Compared with Vitamin K Antagonism for Prevention of Stroke and Embolism Trial in Atrial Fibrillation (ROCKET AF), the authors reported that reduced renal function (creatinine clearances <80 mL/min) had no impact on rivaroxaban's effectiveness and safety [76]. In contrast, a PK/PD study comparing dialysis patients to normal controls reported a 56% increase in AUC when 15 mg doses were administered after dialysis [77]. The AUC was decreased by only 5% when administered pre-dialysis suggesting dialysis is ineffective in clearing the drug [77]. Another PK/PD study comparing three ranges of renal insufficiency to normal controls reported AUCs of 1.4-, 1.5-, and 1.6-fold higher in cases of creatinine clearance concentrations of 50–80, 30–50, and < 30 mL/min, respectively [78].

Pharmacokinetic data for apixaban appear similar to those of rivaroxaban, except that the incremental upsurges in AUC are somewhat lower in magnitude. A small PK/PD study using a 5 mg dose in ESKD patients and normal controls found a 36% increase in AUC in the ESKD group compared to controls. The apixaban dose was administered pre-dialysis [79]. Another small PK/PD study used a single 10 mg dose and compared subjects with varying degrees of CKD to normal controls [8]. Compare to the controls, the AUCs increased by 16%, 29%, and 38% in the CKD cohorts with creatinine clearances of 50–80, 30–50, and < 30 mL/min, respectively. The mean half-life was only slightly increased in the total CKD population (17 h) compared to the controls (15 h) [79]. The overall results for both studies were not unexpected, as apixaban is metabolized more extensively and demonstrates less unchanged renal elimination than other DOACs [1]. Again, the drug appears to be poorly dialyzable [55].

Edoxaban was evaluated in a small PK/PD study comparing CKD subjects to normal controls. The data, available as an abstract only, showed that the mean AUCs increased by 32%, 74%, and 72% with creatinine clearances of 50–80, 30–50, and < 30 mL/min (not on dialysis), respectively [55]. The mean AUC for subjects on peritoneal dialysis was 93% [55]. Similar to other Factor Xa inhibitors, edoxaban is poorly cleared by hemodialysis [80].

Probably, the best data for LMWH come from a subgroup analysis of the ExTRACT TIMI 25 trial. This study compared a 1 mg/kg per day dose of enoxaparin to UFH in ST-elevation myocardial infarction (STEMI) patients with CrCLs less than 30 mL. There was no significant difference in mortality or recurrent MI (33 vs. 37.7%) and in bleeding risk (5.7 vs. 2.8%) for enoxaparin and UFH, respectively. Mortality increased for both drugs as renal function declined [81].

UFH is rapidly eliminated by the reticular endothelial system and, to a lesser extent, the kidney. However, the degree to which the RES functions in this role varies from person to person. Nevertheless, lower doses in VTE treatment are recommended to reduce bleeding risk. An advantage for UFH over enoxaparin is the ability to reverse the former easier with protamine [11, 82].

All DOACs increase AUC with the magnitude inversely proportional to renal function. These drugs may be the anticoagulants of choice for stages 1, 2, and 3 CKD [83]. Some sources recommend apixaban as an alternative to warfarin in selected patients with ESKD [55]. Warfarin, although predominately metabolized in the liver, may require a lower dose to reach a therapeutic INR. Historically, it is the oral anticoagulant of choice in ESKD [11, 82]. However, how does warfarin's potential lack of benefit in ESKD patients with AF apply to PE? Are LMWHs better than UFH? Both were associated with similar mortality increases in STEMI patients with declining kidney function. Should these data also apply to renal failure patients and PE?

9.3 Liver dysfunction

Patients with cirrhosis typically have elevated INR and aPTT. As a result, there have been misconceptions that these patients are "autoanticoagulated." However, patients with liver disease may have a substantially increased risk of VTE (RR 1.74 (95% CI, 1.54–1.95) for liver cirrhosis and 1.87 (95% CI, 1.73–2.03) for non-cirrhotic liver disease) [83]. A meta-analysis in patients with the liver disease found

	Mild impairment (Child-Pugh Class A)	Moderate impairment (Child-Pugh Class B)	Severe impairment (Child-Pugh Class C)
Apixaban	No dosage adjustment.	Use with caution. No dosage adjustments provided.	Use is not recommended.
Rivaroxaban	No dosage adjustment.	Avoid use.	Avoid use.
Edoxaban	No dosage adjustment.	Use is not recommended.	Use is not recommended.
Dabigatran	No dosage adjustment.	Use with caution. No dosage adjustments provided.	No dosage adjustments provided.

Table 3.
FDA recommendations of DOACs in liver dysfunction.

the incidence of PE from nine studies to be 0.28% (95% CI 0.13–0.49%) and the prevalence of PE from two studies to be 0.36% (95% CI 0.13–0.7%) [84].

Determining the ideal anticoagulant to use after a PE in a patient with liver cirrhosis may be challenging. Warfarin can be safely used in patients with liver dysfunction. Elevations in baseline INR due to liver disease, however, may lead to unclear INR targets during warfarin therapy [85, 86]. LMWHs have a good safety profile with liver dysfunction; however, subcutaneous administration may limit compliance, and lower anti-Xa levels in liver dysfunction limit efficacy monitoring [87, 88]. Finally, there are a lack of data on using DOACs in patients with liver disease. Clinical trials with DOACs excluded patients with liver disease as most DOACs are predominantly cleared hepatically (apixaban 75%, rivaroxaban 65%, edoxaban 50%, and dabigatran 20%) [73, 89]. Therefore, dosing recommendations are derived from pharmacokinetic studies (**Table 3**).

Regardless of which anticoagulant is chosen, the risk of bleeding should be thoroughly evaluated. In patients with liver disease, bleeding can be due to varices, portal hypertensive gastropathy, peptic ulcer disease, and arteriovenous malformations. A small, 45-patient cohort study, comparing DOACs to warfarin/LMWH found no difference in thrombotic events. Still, there were significantly fewer major bleeding episodes in the DOAC group (1 patient [4%] vs. 5 patients [28%], p = 0.03) [90].

9.4 Cancer patients

Cancer patients have a five- to sevenfold increased risk for VTE within the first year of diagnosis [91]. Additionally, VTE is considered an independent predictor of mortality in these patients [92, 93]. The pathophysiological and epidemiological association between PE and cancer is well established. For decades, LMWHs were considered a first-line therapy for cancer-associated PEs, as knowledge of the efficacy and safety of DOACs in cancer patients was lacking [77, 94, 95]. Since then, four large randomized control trials have been published comparing DOACs with LMWH that have highlighted the utilization of most DOACs for the treatment of PEs [77, 81, 96, 97].

The Hokusai VTE Cancer trial randomized 1050 cancer patients with acute VTE to either edoxaban, an oral direct factor Xa inhibitor, or dalteparin, an LMWH. The trial found that edoxaban was non-inferior to dalteparin for the primary outcome of recurrent VTE or major bleeding during a follow-up period of 12 months (95% confidence interval 0.70 to 1.36; p = 0.006) [98]. There was a lower rate of VTE, however, nonsignificant risk difference of −3.4 (−7.0 to 0.2), but the major bleeding rate was significantly higher (risk difference of 2.9 (0.1 to 5.6)) [98]. A nonsignificant lower VTE rate was seen, but the major bleeding rate was significantly higher in the edoxaban group. Major bleeding events were frequently observed in the subgroup with upper gastrointestinal tract neoplasms [98].

SELECT-D randomized 406 patients with cancer and acute VTE to oral rivaroxaban, a factor, or dalteparin for a treatment duration of 6 months [99]. SELECT-D was a 6-month open-label, pilot, randomized control study that compared rivaroxaban 15 mg BID for 3 weeks then 20 mg once daily to dalteparin (200 IU/kg once daily for 1 month, then 150 IU/kg once daily) in patients with VTE and solid or hematologic cancers [99]. The trial found that the VTE recurrence rate was 4% with rivaroxaban and 11% with dalteparin (HR 0.43, 95% CI 0.19 to 0.99) [99]. Major bleeding occurred in 4% with dalteparin and 6% with rivaroxaban (HR 1.83, 95% CI 0.68 to 4.96) and clinically relevant, nonmajor bleeding occurred in 4% with dalteparin and 13% with rivaroxaban (HR 3.76, 95% 1.63 to 8.69) [99].

CARAVAGGIO was an open-label, non-inferior study that randomized 1170 patients to apixaban (10 mg twice daily for 7 days, then 5 mg twice daily) or dalteparin (200 IU/kg once daily for 1 month, then 150 IU/kg once daily) for 6 months of treatment [100]. The trial resulted in a VTE recurrence rate of 5.6% with apixaban and 7.9% with dalteparin (risk difference − 2.3%; HR 0.63, 95% CI 0.37 to 1.07, $p < 0.001$) [100]. Additionally, major bleeding occurred in 3.8% in the apixaban group versus 4% in the dalteparin group (risk difference − 0.2%; HR 0.82, 95% CI 0.4 to 1.69, $p = 0.60$) [100].

Given that these oral agents have shown efficacy and provide a more convenient medication dosage form, we have already begun to see a shift in the way PEs are treated in cancer patients [77, 81, 96, 97]. However, since many of these studies have excluded patients with GI tumors or a history of GI bleeding, it is still recommended to continue using LMWH in these patients due to the higher GI bleeding risk seen with DOACs [77, 81, 96, 97]. If a DOAC is to be utilized, the choice of which oral anticoagulant to be used in a cancer patient should be made on an individual basis with considerations of drug interactions with chemotherapy agents and the type of cancer.

9.5 Pregnancy

UFH and LMWH remain the only currently available choices for the safe management of VTE including PE during pregnancy and puerperium. UFH provides the least exposure to the fetus and risk to the mother, since it does not cross the placenta, is not distributed into breast milk, and the dose is easily titrated [101]. LMWHs have a similar safety profile as UFH for the fetus since they also do not cross the placenta. Concerns about distribution into breast milk have been raised [101, 102]. Most studies have not demonstrated that the LMWH levels in breast milk are high enough to cause coagulopathy when using standard prophylaxis doses. Further studies are needed for a complete safety profile.

The ability to easily monitor aPPT levels for UFH and anti-Xa levels for LMWHs provides clinicians with the ability to maintain therapeutic concentrations throughout pregnancy. Therapeutic-level monitoring provides safety and efficacy for both the fetus and the mother, since changes in the drug volume of distribution and clearance progressively increase throughout pregnancy [23, 101, 103–105]. Additionally, UFH and LMWH have short half-lives, allowing for anticoagulation to be maintained within 24 h of delivery and permitting the safe use of neuroaxial anesthesia if needed [102, 106]. Restarting LMWH within 6 h postdelivery in patients without bleeding concerns has been shown to be safe. Anticoagulation should be maintained during puerperium [101]. Thromboprophylaxis for future pregnancies with UFH or LMWH is recommended for women at risk [107, 108].

The safety profile and pharmacokinetics of DOACs currently do not favor their use during pregnancy or puerperium, since they cross the placenta and distribute into breast milk [101, 109]. The use of DOACs may be considered in women who are not or are no longer breastfeeding. The inability to readily monitor DOAC levels limits the clinician's ability to maintain therapeutic levels throughout pregnancy and puerperium due to the pharmacokinetic changes listed above. Maintaining a safe and therapeutic efficacious anticoagulation regimen up to and through the time of delivery requires a multidisciplinary effort and needs to be closely coordinated [101, 102, 106].

9.6 Elderly

The risk of thromboembolic disease, including PE, increases with age [110–112]. The trauma to the vascular endothelium caused by a thromboembolic event places the patient at a higher risk of recurrence, requiring prolonged anticoagulation [110, 113]. Comorbidities accompanying aging, especially cardiovascular and pulmonary disease, add to the complexity of treatment of thromboembolic disease [114]. The increased risk for bleeding further complicates the safe management of an acute venous thromboembolic event, and prolonged anticoagulation is required to prevent future events [4].

PE in elderly patients may not present with the typical symptoms seen in younger patients, making early diagnosis more challenging in this population. Several studies have found syncope to be the most frequent presenting symptom in elderly patients, versus pleuritic chest pain in a younger population [115–117]. Early pharmacotherapy intervention is critical to prevent further thrombus formation, regardless of the patient's age [110].

Recommendations for initial treatment for PE in a stable patient regardless of the prognosis include DOACs (apixaban or rivaroxaban) or initial LMWH, followed with dabigatran or edoxaban. LMWH or UFH and warfarin may be preferred in patients with reduced renal function (CrCL <30 mL/min) [118].

Stable patients with a good prognosis may be managed in an outpatient setting. The current recommendations for stable patients with a poor prognosis require hospitalization [118]. A thorough medication history is important prior to starting a DOAC due to the potential drug–drug interactions seen with this class of anticoagulants. P-glycoprotein inhibitors or CYP3A4 inhibitors or inducers should be avoided, since they can alter the plasma of DOACs [118]. The unstable patient requires hospitalization and may be a candidate for thrombolytic therapy, preferably by catheter-directed thrombolysis [118].

9.7 COVID-19 patients

The emergence of severe acute respiratory syndrome coronavirus 2 (SARS-CoV-2) from Wuhan, Hubei province, China, in December 2019 has adversely impacted the world. Among the several complications related to SARS-CoV-2 is VTE [119], a systematic review of 3487 COVID-19 patients from 30 studies demonstrated VTE incidence to be 26%, 12% for PE with or without DVT, and 14% for DVT alone.

The etiology of PE in COVID-19 is secondary to the well-known VTE risk factors, with indirect aspects of the severity of illness and direct effects of SARS-CoV2 viral infection. These patients are at VTE risk due to the recurrent use of intravascular access devices, sedation, and vasopressors, within the intensive care unit (ICU) setting. These factors promote stasis. Respiratory failure, hypoxia, comorbidities, multi-organ failure, obesity, and prolonged immobility are other elements. Additional confounding factors include a history of VTE and or neoplasm, sepsis, surgery, trauma, or stroke [120, 121].

COVID-19 is associated with a profound early response of proinflammatory cytokines. This may result in a cytokine storm, increased risk of vascular hyperpermeability, multi-organ failure, and death [122, 123]. While thrombin's primary role is to accelerate clot formation *via* platelet activation and the conversion of fibrinogen to fibrin, thrombin equally exerts multiple cellular effects. It could further enhance inflammation through proteinase-activated receptors (PARs). Thrombin production is highly regulated *via* negative feedback mechanisms and physiological anticoagulants, such as the protein C system, antithrombin III, and tissue factor pathway inhibitor [124]. These three control mechanisms may become impaired throughout the inflammatory process, resulting in decreased anticoagulant concentrations secondary to reduced production and increased consumption. This impaired procoagulant–anticoagulant equilibrium results in disseminated intravascular coagulation (DIC), microthrombosis, multi-organ failure, and elevated d-dimer levels [91, 125, 126]. Hypercoagulable state, endothelial dysfunction, injury, and viral-induced procoagulant effect all also play an immense role in COVID-19-associated PE [127–129].

Both LMWH and UFH are recommended for VTE prophylaxis and PE treatment in COVID-19 patients. The recommended dose of the LMWH enoxaparin for VTE prophylaxis is 40 mg (4000 IU) daily. An intermediate dose of LMWH enoxaparin 40 mg subcutaneously every 12 h is recommended in the critically ill, the obese, and those patients with multiple VTE risk factors. A UFH dose of 5000 IU Q8H is recommended for VTE prophylaxis, and doses of up to 7500 IU have been employed in critically ill patients [98–100, 130, 131]. DOACs are recommended in stable patients and in the post-acute phase of PE and outpatient settings when the benefits from their use outweigh the risks. Renal function monitoring with dosage modifications is recommended when LMWH, UFH, and DOACs are employed. Additionally, Anti-Xa monitoring is recommended in patients requiring the therapeutic anticoagulation with LMWH, UFH, and DOAC therapy. DOAC plasma level monitoring is also recommended [101, 131]. Therapeutic anticoagulation should always be considered first; thrombolytic therapy is recommended in patients who go to develop sub-massive or massive PE. An inferior vena cava filter may be employed in at-risk patients; extracorporeal membrane oxygenator (ECMO) is an option, in conjunction with surgical embolectomy or catheter-directed management [1, 102, 103]. Several weeks of therapy is recommended with LMWH or DOACs, post-hospitalization for COVID-19 patients [132].

10. Conclusions

PE is a medical emergency that affects thousands of Americans each year. Thousands of Americans die from this condition annually. The therapy for PE has evolved over the years. Traditional therapies such as UFH, VKA, and warfarin are being abandoned by clinicians in favor of LMWH and DOACs. Reversal agents such as 4-factor prothrombin complex concentrate, andaxanet alfa, and the monoclonal antibody idarucizumab have allowed clinicians to push the boundaries of PE management with confidence, particularly in the outpatient setting. Special populations, such as obese, renal dysfunction, liver impairment, cancer, pregnancy, and COVID-19 patients with PE, pose a tremendous therapeutic burden and challenge to clinicians. Despite these challenges, tremendous progress has been made, with demonstrated improved patient outcomes in PE treatment over the last three decades.

Conflict of interest

The authors declare no conflict of interest.

Author details

Ladan Panahi, George Udeani*, Michael Horseman, Jaye Weston, Nephy Samuel, Merlyn Joseph, Andrea Mora, Daniela Bazan and Pooja Patel
Department of Pharmacy Practice, Texas A&M Rangel College of Pharmacy, Kingsville, USA and College Station, Texas, USA

*Address all correspondence to: udeani@tamu.edu

IntechOpen

References

[1] Essien EO, Rali P, Mathai SC. Pulmonary embolism. Medical Clinics of North America. 2019;**103**:549-564

[2] Girard P, Decousus M, Laporte S, Buchmuller A, Hervé Philippe; Lamer C; Parent F; Tardy B. Diagnosis of pulmonary embolism in patients with proximal deep vein thrombosis: Specificity of symptoms and perfusion defects at baseline and during anticoagulant therapy. American Journal of Respiratory and Critical Care Medicine. 2001;**164**:1033-1037

[3] Di Nisio M, van Es N, Büller HR. Deep vein thrombosis and pulmonary embolism. Lancet. 2016;**388**:3060-3073

[4] Kearon C, Akl EA, Ornelas J, Blaivas A, Jimenez D, Bounameaux H, et al. Antithrombotic therapy for VTE disease: CHEST guideline and expert panel report. Chest. 2016;**149**:315-352

[5] Kahn SR, Lim W, Dunn AS, Cushman M, Dentali F, Akl EA, et al. Prevention of VTE in nonsurgical patients: Antithrombotic therapy and prevention of thrombosis: American College of Chest Physicians evidence-based clinical practice guidelines. Chest. 2012;**2012**(*141*):e195S-e226S

[6] FDA Highlights of Prescribing Information Unfractionated Heparin. Available online: https://www.accessdata.fda.gov/drugsatfda_docs/label/2017/017029s140lbl.pdf [Accessed: 21 October 2020].

[7] Garcia DA, Baglin TP, Weitz JI, Samama MM. Parenteral anticoagulants: Antithrombotic therapy and prevention of thrombosis, 9th ed: American College of Chest Physicians Evidence-Based Clinical Practice Guidelines. Chest. 2012;**141**(Suppl. 2):e24S-e43S

[8] Smythe MA, Priziola J, Dobesh PP, Wirth D, Cuker A, Wittkowsky AK. Guidance for the practical management of the heparin anticoagulants in the treatment of venous thromboembolism. Journal of Thrombosis and Thrombolysis. 2016;**41**:165-186

[9] Sebaaly J, Covert K. Enoxaparin dosing at extremes of weight: Literature review and dosing recommendations. The Annals of Pharmacotherapy. 2018;**52**:898-909

[10] Insert P. *Fragmin (Dalteparin Sodium)*. Peapack, NJ, USA: Pharmacia Peapack; 2020

[11] Squibb B-M. *Eliquis (Apixaban) Package Insert*. Princeton, NJ, USA: Bristol-Myers Squibb; 2014

[12] Pharmaceuticals J. *Xarelto (Rivaroxaban) Package Insert*. Beerse, Belgium: Janssen Pharmaceuticals Inc.; 2020

[13] Mueck W, Stampfuss J, Kubitza D, Becka M. Clinical pharmacokinetic and pharmacodynamic profile of rivaroxaban. Clinical Pharmacokinetics. 2014;**53**:1-16

[14] Shah A, Crawford D, Burger D, Martin N, Walker M, Talley NJ, et al. Effects of antibiotic therapy in primary sclerosing cholangitis with and without inflammatory bowel disease: A systematic review and meta-analysis. Seminars in Liver Disease. 2019;**39**:432-441

[15] Byon W, Garonzik S, Boyd RA, Frost CE. Apixaban: A clinical pharmacokinetic and pharmacodynamic review. Clinical Pharmacokinetics. Oct;**58**(10):1265-1279

[16] Boehringer Ingelheim Pharmaceuticals. *Pradaxa (Dabigatran) Package Insert*. Ridgefield, CT, USA: Boehringer Ingelheim; 2020

[17] Salter BS, Weiner MM, Trinh MA, Heller J, Evans AS, Adams DH, et al. Heparin-induced thrombocytopenia: A comprehensive clinical Review. Journal of the American College of Cardiology. 2016;**67**:2519-2532

[18] Cuker A, Arepally GM, Chong BH, Cines DB, Greinacher A, Gruel Y, et al. American Society of Hematology 2018 guidelines for management of venous thromboembolism: Heparin-induced thrombocytopenia. Blood Advances. 2018;**2**:3360-3392

[19] Mahan CE, Spyropoulos AC. ASHP therapeutic position statement on the role of pharmacotherapy in preventing venous thromboembolism in hospitalized patients. American Journal of Health-System Pharmacy. 2012;**69**:2174-2190

[20] Linkins LA, Dans AL, Moores LK, Bona R, Davidson BL, Schulman S, et al. Treatment and prevention of heparin-induced thrombocytopenia: Antithrombotic therapy and prevention of thrombosis: American College of Chest Physicians evidence-based clinical practice guidelines. Chest. 2012;**141**: e495S-e530S

[21] Hirsh J, Warkentin TE, Shaughnessy SG, Anand SS, Halperin JL, Raschke R, et al. Heparin and low-molecular-weight heparin mechanisms of action, pharmacokinetics, dosing, monitoring, efficacy, and safety. Chest. 2001;**119**: 64S-94S

[22] Hirsh J, Lee AY. How we diagnose and treat deep vein thrombosis. Blood, the flagship journal of the American Society of Hematology. 2002;**99**: 3102-3110

[23] Duffett L, Castellucci LA, Forgie MA. Pulmonary embolism: Update on management and controversies. BMJ. 2020;**5**:370

[24] Sallah S, Thomas DP, Roberts HR. Warfarin and heparin-induced skin necrosis and the purple toe syndrome: Infrequent complications of anticoagulant treatment. Thrombosis and Haemostasis. 1997;**78**:785-790

[25] Guyatt GH, Akl EA, Crowther M, Gutterman DD, Schuünemann HJ. Executive summary: Antithrombotic therapy and prevention of thrombosis: American College of Chest Physicians evidence-based clinical practice guidelines. Chest. 2012;**141**(Suppl. 2):7S

[26] Squibb B-M. *Coumadin (Warfarin) Package Insert*. Princeton, NJ, USA: Bristol-Myers Squibb; 2019

[27] Ansell J, Hirsh J, Hylek E, Jacobson A, Crowther M, Palareti G. Pharmacology and management of the vitamin K antagonists: American College of Chest Physicians evidence-based clinical practice guidelines. Chest. 2008;**133**:160S-198S

[28] Ageno W, Gallus AS, Wittkowsky A, Crowther M, Hylek EM, Palareti G. Oral anticoagulant therapy: Antithrombotic therapy and prevention of thrombosis: American College of Chest Physicians evidence-based clinical practice guidelines. Chest. 2012;**141**:e44S-e88S

[29] Tomaselli GF, Mahaffey KW, Cuker A, Dobesh PP, Doherty JU, Eikelboom JW, et al. 2020 ACC expert consensus decision pathway on management of bleeding in patients on oral anticoagulants: A report of the American College of Cardiology Solution Set Oversight Committee. Journal of the American College of Cardiology. 2020;**76**:594-622

[30] UW Medicine. Guidelines for Reversal of Anticoagulants. 2020. Available from: https://depts. washington.edu/anticoag/home/sites/ default/files/GUIDELINES%20 FOR%20REVERSAL%20OF%20 ANTICOAGULANTS.pdf [Accessed: 19 October 2020]

[31] Insert MILP. *Arixtra (Fondaparinux Sodium) Injection*. Rockford, IL, USA: Mylan Institutional LLC Package; 2017

[32] Yee J, Kaide CG. Emergency Reversal of Anticoagulation. The Western Journal of Emergency Medicine. 2019;**20**:770-783

[33] Wang L, Zhang D, Raghavan N, Yao M, Ma L, Frost CA, et al. In vitro assessment of metabolic drug-drug interaction potential of apixaban through cytochrome P450 phenotyping, inhibition, and induction studies. Drug Metabolism and Disposition. 2010;**38**:448-458

[34] Lopes RD, Heizer G, Aronson R, Vora AN, Massaro T, Mehran R, et al. Antithrombotic therapy after acute coronary syndrome or PCI in atrial fibrillation. The New England Journal of Medicine. 2019;**380**:1509-1524

[35] Barlow A, Barlow B, Reinaker T, Harris J. Potential role of direct oral anticoagulants in the management of heparin-induced thrombocytopenia. Pharmacotherapy: The Journal of Human Pharmacology and Drug Therapy. 2019;**39**:837-853

[36] I Pp. *Andexxa (coagulation Factor Xa (Recombinant), Inactivated-Zhzo): US Prescribing Information*. San Francisco, CA, USA: Portola pharmaceuticals Inc.; 2018

[37] Liu Y, Xu S. Post-conditioning the human heart: Technical concerns beyond the protocol algorithm. Journal of the American College of Cardiology. 2013;**62**:1216-1217

[38] Kim IS, Kim HJ, Yu HT, Kim TH, Uhm JS, Kim JY, et al. Non-vitamin K antagonist oral anticoagulants with amiodarone, P-glycoprotein inhibitors, or polypharmacy in patients with atrial fibrillation: Systematic review and meta-analysis. Journal of Cardiology. 2019;**73**:515-521

[39] Vazquez SR. Drug-drug interactions in an era of multiple anticoagulants: A focus on clinically relevant drug interactions. Hematology. American Society of Hematology. Education Program. 2018;**2018**:339-347

[40] Zhang D, He K, Herbst JJ, Kolb J, Shou W, Wang L, et al. Characterization of efflux transporters involved in distribution and disposition of apixaban. Drug Metabolism and Disposition. 2013;**41**:827-835

[41] By the American Geriatrics Society Beers Criteria Update Expert P. American Geriatrics Society. Updated AGS beers criteria(R) for potentially inappropriate medication use in older adults. Journal of the American Geriatrics Society. 2019;**2019**(67): 674-694

[42] Eikelboom JW, Connolly SJ, Brueckmann M, Granger CB, Kappetein AP, Mack MJ, et al. Dabigatran versus warfarin in patients with mechanical heart valves. The New England Journal of Medicine. 2013;**369**:1206-1214

[43] Kim JS, Lee HJ, Sung JD, Kim H-J, Lee S-Y, Kim JS. Monitoring of unfractionated heparin using activated partial thromboplastin time: An assessment of the current nomogram and analysis according to age. Clinical and Applied Thrombosis/Hemostasis. 2014;**20**:723-728

[44] Investigators H-VTE. Edoxaban versus warfarin for the treatment of symptomatic venous thromboembolism. The New England Journal of Medicine. 2013;**369**:1406-1415

[45] Daiichi Sankyo Co. *Savaysa (Edoxaban) [Package Insert]*. Tokyo, Japan: Daiichi Sankyo Co.; 2015

[46] Stacy ZA, Call WB, Hartmann AP, Peters GL, Richter SK. Edoxaban: A comprehensive review of the

pharmacology and clinical data for the management of atrial fibrillation and venous thromboembolism. Cardiology and Therapy. 2016;**5**:1-18

[47] Hao Q, Dong BR, Yue J, Wu T, Liu GJ. Thrombolytic therapy for pulmonary embolism. Cochrane Database of Systematic Reviews. 2018 Dec 18;**12**(12):1-101

[48] Konstantinides SV, Meyer G, Becattini C, Bueno H, Geersing GJ, Harjola VP, et al. 2019 ESC Guidelines for the diagnosis and management of acute pulmonary embolism developed in collaboration with the European Respiratory Society (ERS) The Task Force for the diagnosis and management of acute pulmonary embolism of the European Society of Cardiology (ESC). European Heart Journal. 2020;**41**: 543-603

[49] Meneveau N, Seronde MF, Blonde MC, Legalery P, Didier-Petit K, Briand F, et al. Management of unsuccessful thrombolysis in acute massive pulmonary embolism. Chest. 2006;**129**:1043-1050

[50] Konstantinides S, Tiede N, Geibel A, Olschewski M, Just H, Kasper W. Comparison of alteplase versus heparin for resolution of major pulmonary embolism. The American Journal of Cardiology. 1998;**82**:966-970

[51] Malik S, Bhardwaj A, Eisen M, Gandhi S. Advanced management options for massive and submassive pulmonary embolism. US Cardiology Review. 2016;**10**:30-35

[52] White RH. The epidemiology of venous thromboembolism. Circulation. 2003;**107**(Suppl. 1):I-4-I-8

[53] Meyer G, Vicaut E, Danays T, Agnelli G, Becattini C, Beyer-Westendorf J, et al. Fibrinolysis for patients with intermediate-risk pulmonary embolism. The New England Journal of Medicine. 2014;**370**:1402-1411

[54] Saborido CM, Jimenez D, Muriel A, Zamora J, Morillo R, Barrios DD, et al. Efficacy and safety outcomes of recanalization procedures in patients with acute symptomatic pulmonary embolism: Systematic review And network meta-analysis. Value in Health. 2017;**20**:A604-A605

[55] Ortel TL, Neumann I, Ageno W, Beyth R, Clark NP, Cuker A, et al. American Society of Hematology 2020 guidelines for management of venous thromboembolism: Treatment of deep vein thrombosis and pulmonary embolism. Blood Advances. 2020;**4**:4693-4738

[56] Brandt K, McGinn K, Quedado J. Low-dose systemic alteplase (tPA) for the treatment of pulmonary embolism. The Annals of Pharmacotherapy. 2015;**49**:818-824

[57] St Pierre BP, Edwin SB. Assessment of anticoagulation in patients receiving ultrasound-assisted catheter-directed thrombolysis for treatment of pulmonary embolism. The Annals of Pharmacotherapy. 2019;**53**:453-457

[58] Kearon C, Akl EA, Comerota AJ, Prandoni P, Bounameaux H, Goldhaber SZ, et al. Antithrombotic therapy for VTE disease: Antithrombotic therapy and prevention of thrombosis: American College of Chest Physicians evidence-based clinical practice guidelines. Chest. 2012;**141**:e419S-e496S

[59] Kline JA, Hernandez-Nino J, Jones AE. Tenecteplase to treat pulmonary embolism in the emergency department. Journal of Thrombosis and Thrombolysis. 2007;**23**:101-105

[60] Holbrook A, Schulman S, Witt DM, Vandvik PO, Fish J, Kovacs MJ, et al. Evidence-based management of anticoagulant therapy: Antithrombotic therapy and prevention of thrombosis: American College of Chest Physicians evidence-based clinical practice guidelines. Chest. 2012;**141**:e152S-e184S

[61] Vandiver JW, Vondracek TG. Antifactor Xa levels versus activated partial thromboplastin time for monitoring unfractionated heparin. Pharmacotherapy: The Journal of Human Pharmacology and Drug Therapy. 2012;**32**:546-558

[62] Guervil DJ, Rosenberg AF, Winterstein AG, Harris NS, Johns TE, Zumberg MS. Activated partial thromboplastin time versus antifactor Xa heparin assay in monitoring unfractionated heparin by continuous intravenous infusion. The Annals of Pharmacotherapy. 2011;**45**:861-868

[63] Bussey HI. Problems with monitoring heparin anticoagulation. Pharmacotherapy: The Journal of Human Pharmacology and Drug Therapy. 1999;**19**:2-5

[64] Francis JL, Groce IIIJB, Group H.C. Challenges in variation and responsiveness of unfractionated heparin. Pharmacotherapy: The Journal of Human Pharmacology and Drug Therapy. 2004;**24**:108S-119S

[65] Olson JD, Arkin CF, Brandt JT, Cunningham T, Giles A, Koepke JA, et al. College of American Pathologists Conference XXXI on laboratory monitoring of anticoagulant therapy. Archives of Pathology & Laboratory Medicine. 1998;**122**:782-798

[66] Frugé KS, Lee YR. Comparison of unfractionated heparin protocols using antifactor Xa monitoring or activated partial thrombin time monitoring. American Journal of Health-System Pharmacy. 2015;**72**(Suppl. 2):S90-S97

[67] Byun J-H, Jang I-S, Kim JW, Koh E-H. Establishing the heparin therapeutic range using aPTT and anti-Xa measurements for monitoring unfractionated heparin therapy. Blood Research. 2016;**51**:171-174

[68] Smith ML, Wheeler KE. Weight-based heparin protocol using antifactor Xa monitoring. American Journal of Health-System Pharmacy. 2010;**67**: 371-374

[69] Riney JN, Hollands JM, Smith JR, Deal EN. Identifying optimal initial infusion rates for unfractionated heparin in morbidly obese patients. The Annals of Pharmacotherapy. 2010;**44**:1141-1151

[70] Arachchillage D, Kamani F, Deplano S, Banya W, Laffan M. Should we abandon the APTT for monitoring unfractionated heparin? Thrombosis Research. 2017;**157**:157-161

[71] Graves KK, Edholm K, Johnson SA. Use of oral anticoagulants in obese patients. JSM Atherosclerosis. 2017;**2**:1035

[72] Rizk E, Wilson AD, Murillo MU, Putney DR. Comparison of antifactor Xa and activated partial thromboplastin time monitoring for heparin dosing in vascular surgery patients: A single-center retrospective study. Therapeutic Drug Monitoring. 2018;**40**:151-155

[73] Owen RP, Gong L, Sagreiya H, Klein TE, Altman RB. VKORC1 pharmacogenomics summary. Pharmacogenetics and Genomics. 2010;**20**:642-644

[74] Connolly SJ, Ezekowitz MD, Yusuf S, Eikelboom J, Oldgren J, Parekh A, et al. Dabigatran versus warfarin in patients with atrial fibrillation. The New England Journal of Medicine. 2009;**361**:1139-1151

[75] Schulman S, Kearon C, Kakkar AK, Mismetti P, Schellong S, Eriksson H, et al. Dabigatran versus warfarin in the treatment of acute venous thromboembolism. The New England Journal of Medicine. 2009;**361**: 2342-2352

[76] Breuer L, Ringwald J, Schwab S, Kohrmann M. Ischemic stroke in an

obese patient receiving dabigatran. The New England Journal of Medicine. 2013;**368**:2440-2442

[77] Dias C, Moore KT, Murphy J, Ariyawansa J, Smith W, Mills RM, et al. Pharmacokinetics, pharmacodynamics, and safety of single-dose rivaroxaban in chronic hemodialysis. American Journal of Nephrology. 2016;**43**: 229-236

[78] Kubitza D, Becka M, Mueck W, Zuehlsdorf M. Safety, tolerability, pharmacodynamics, and pharmacokinetics of rivaroxaban--an oral, direct factor Xa inhibitor--are not affected by aspirin. Journal of Clinical Pharmacology. 2006;**46**:981-990

[79] Mueck W, Lensing AW, Agnelli G, Decousus H, Prandoni P, Misselwitz F. Rivaroxaban: Population pharmacokinetic analyses in patients treated for acute deep-vein thrombosis and exposure simulations in patients with atrial fibrillation treated for stroke prevention. Clinical Pharmacokinetics. 2011;**50**:675-686

[80] Upreti VV, Wang J, Barrett YC, Byon W, Boyd RA, Pursley J, et al. Effect of extremes of body weight on the pharmacokinetics, pharmacodynamics, safety and tolerability of apixaban in healthy subjects. British Journal of Clinical Pharmacology. 2013;**76**: 908-916

[81] Fox KA, Antman EM, Montalescot G, Agewall S, SomaRaju B, Verheugt FW, et al. The impact of renal dysfunction on outcomes in the ExTRACT-TIMI 25 trial. Journal of the American College of Cardiology. 2007;**49**:2249-2255

[82] Granger CB, Alexander JH, McMurray JJ, Lopes RD, Hylek EM, Hanna M, et al. Apixaban versus warfarin in patients with atrial fibrillation. The New England Journal of Medicine. 2011;**365**:981-992

[83] Sogaard KK, Horvath-Puho E, Gronbaek H, Jepsen P, Vilstrup H, Sorensen HT. Risk of venous thromboembolism in patients with liver disease: A nationwide population-based case-control study. The American Journal of Gastroenterology. 2009;**104**:96-101

[84] Qi X, Ren W, Guo X, Fan D. Epidemiology of venous thromboembolism in patients with liver diseases: A systematic review and meta-analysis. Internal and Emergency Medicine. 2015;**10**:205-217

[85] Shlensky JA, Thurber KM, O'Meara JG, Ou NN, Osborn JL, Dierkhising RA, et al. Unfractionated heparin infusion for treatment of venous thromboembolism based on actual body weight without dose capping. Vascular Medicine. 2020;**25**:47-54

[86] Witt DM, Nieuwlaat R, Clark NP, Ansell J, Holbrook A, Skov J, et al. American Society of Hematology 2018 guidelines for management of venous thromboembolism: Optimal management of anticoagulation therapy. Blood Advances. 2018;**2**:3257-3291

[87] Jain N, Reilly RF. Clinical pharmacology of oral anticoagulants in patients with kidney disease. Clinical Journal of the American Society of Nephrology. 2019;**14**:278-287

[88] Harder S. Renal profiles of anticoagulants. Journal of Clinical Pharmacology. 2012;**52**:964-975

[89] Limdi NA, Beasley TM, Baird MF, Goldstein JA, McGwin G, Arnett DK, et al. Kidney function influences warfarin responsiveness and hemorrhagic complications. Journal of the American Society of Nephrology. 2009;**20**:912-921

[90] Limdi NA, Limdi MA, Cavallari L, Anderson AM, Crowley MR, Baird MF, et al. Warfarin dosing in patients with

impaired kidney function. American Journal of Kidney Diseases. 2010;**56**: 823-831

[91] Ella I, Tapson VF. Advances in the diagnosis of acute pulmonary embolism. F1000Res. 2020 Jan 24;**9**:F1000 Faculty Rev-44

[92] Randhawa MS, Vishwanath R, Rai MP, Wang L, Randhawa AK, Abela G, et al. Association between use of warfarin for atrial fibrillation and outcomes among patients with end-stage renal disease: A systematic review and meta-analysis. JAMA Network Open. 2020;**3**:e202175

[93] Stangier J, Rathgen K, Stahle H, Mazur D. Influence of renal impairment on the pharmacokinetics and pharmacodynamics of oral dabigatran etexilate: An open-label, parallel-group, single-centre study. Clinical Pharmacokinetics. 2010;**49**:259-268

[94] Hori M, Matsumoto M, Tanahashi N, Momomura SI, Uchiyama S, Goto S, et al. Rivaroxaban vs. warfarin in Japanese patients with atrial fibrillation—The J-ROCKET AF study. Circulation Journal. 2012;**76**:2104-2111

[95] Kubitza D, Becka M, Mueck W, Halabi A, Maatouk H, Klause N, et al. Effects of renal impairment on the pharmacokinetics, pharmacodynamics and safety of rivaroxaban, an oral, direct Factor Xa inhibitor. British Journal of Clinical Pharmacology. 2010;**70**:703-712

[96] Chang M, Yu Z, Shenker A, Wang J, Pursley J, Byon W, et al. Effect of renal impairment on the pharmacokinetics, pharmacodynamics, and safety of apixaban. Journal of Clinical Pharmacology. 2016;**56**:637-645

[97] Parasrampuria DA, Marbury T, Matsushima N, Chen S, Wickremasingha PK, He L, et al. Pharmacokinetics, safety, and tolerability of edoxaban in end-stage renal disease subjects undergoing haemodialysis. Thrombosis and Haemostasis. 2015;**113**:719-727

[98] Raskob GE, van Es N, Verhamme P, Carrier M, Di Nisio M, Garcia D, et al. Edoxaban for the treatment of cancer-associated venous thromboembolism. The New England Journal of Medicine. 2018;**378**:615-624

[99] Young AM, Marshall A, Thirlwall J, Chapman O, Lokare A, Hill C, et al. Comparison of an oral factor Xa inhibitor with low molecular weight heparin in patients with cancer with venous thromboembolism: Results of a randomized trial (SELECT-D). J Clin Oncol. 2018 Jul 10;**36**(20):2017-2023.

[100] Agnelli G, Becattini C, Meyer G, Muñoz A, Huisman MV, Connors JM, et al. Apixaban for the treatment of venous thromboembolism associated with cancer. The New England Journal of Medicine. 2020;**382**:1599-1607

[101] Lim W, Le Gal G, Bates SM, Righini M, Haramati LB, Lang E, et al. American Society of Hematology 2018 guidelines for management of venous thromboembolism: Venous thromboembolism in the context of pregnancy. Blood Advances. 2018;**2**:3317-3359

[102] Richter C, Sitzmann J, Lang P, Weitzel H, Huch A, Huch R. Excretion of low molecular weight heparin in human milk. British Journal of Clinical Pharmacology. 2001;**52**:708-710

[103] Costantine M. Physiologic and pharmacokinetic changes in pregnancy. Frontiers in Pharmacology. 2014;**5**:65

[104] Pariente G, Leibson T, Carls A, Adams-Webber T, Ito S, Koren G. Pregnancy-associated changes in pharmacokinetics: A systematic review. PLoS Medicine. 2016;**13**:e1002160

[105] Davis M, Simmons C, Dordoni B, Maxwell J, Williams R. Induction of hepatic enzymes during normal human pregnancy. BJOG: An International Journal of Obstetrics & Gynaecology. 1973;**80**:690-694

[106] Gogarten W, Vandermeulen E, Van Aken H, Kozek S, Llau JV, Samama CM. Regional anaesthesia and antithrombotic agents: Recommendations of the European Society of Anaesthesiology. The European Journal of Anaesthesiology (EJA). 2010;**27**:999-1015

[107] Horlocker TT, Vandermeuelen E, Kopp SL, Gogarten W, Leffert LR, Benzon HT. Regional anesthesia in the patient receiving antithrombotic or thrombolytic therapy: American Society of Regional Anesthesia and Pain Medicine Evidence-Based Guidelines. Obstetric Anesthesia Digest. 2019;**39**: 28-29

[108] Lameijer H, Aalberts JJ, van Veldhuisen DJ, Meijer K, Pieper PG. Efficacy and safety of direct oral anticoagulants during pregnancy; a systematic literature review. Thrombosis Research. 2018;**169**:123-127

[109] Bapat P, Pinto LSR, Lubetsky A, Berger H, Koren G. Rivaroxaban transfer across the dually perfused isolated human placental cotyledon. American Journal of Obstetrics and Gynecology. 2015;**213**:e1-e710

[110] Robert-Ebadi H, Righini M. Diagnosis and management of pulmonary embolism in the elderly. European Journal of Internal Medicine. 2014;**25**:343-349

[111] Silverstein MD, Heit JA, Mohr DN, Petterson TM, O'Fallon WM, Melton LJ. Trends in the incidence of deep vein thrombosis and pulmonary embolism: A 25-year population-based study. Archives of Internal Medicine. 1998;**158**:585-593

[112] Anderson FA, Wheeler HB, Goldberg RJ, Hosmer DW, Forcier A. A population-based perspective of the hospital incidence and case-fatality rates of deep vein thrombosis and pulmonary embolism: The Worcester DVT Study. Archives of Internal Medicine. 1991;**151**:933-938

[113] Goldhaber SZ, Visani L, De Rosa M. Acute pulmonary embolism: Clinical outcomes in the International Cooperative Pulmonary Embolism Registry (ICOPER). Lancet. 1999;**353**: 1386-1389

[114] Stein PD, Matta F. Treatment of unstable pulmonary embolism in the elderly and those with comorbid conditions. The American Journal of Medicine. 2013;**126**:304-310

[115] Tisserand G, Gil H, Méaux-Ruault N, Magy-Bertrand N. Clinical features of pulmonary embolism in elderly: A comparative study of 64 patients. La Revue de Médecine Interne. 2014;**35**:353-356

[116] Timmons S, Kingston M, Hussain M, Kelly H, Liston R. Pulmonary embolism: Differences in presentation between older and younger patients. Age and Ageing. 2003;**32**:601-605

[117] Kokturk N, Oguzulgen IK, Demir N, Demirel K, Ekim N. Differences in clinical presentation of pulmonary embolism in older vs younger patients. Circulation Journal. 2005;**69**:981-986

[118] Tritschler T, Kraaijpoel N, Le Gal G, Wells PS. Venous thromboembolism: Advances in diagnosis and treatment. JAMA. 2018;**320**:1583-1594

[119] Terpos E, Ntanasis-Stathopoulos I, Elalamy I, Kastritis E, Sergentanis TN, Politou M, et al. Hematological findings and complications of COVID-19. American Journal of Hematology. 2020;**213**:e1-e710

[120] Buresi M, Hull R, Coffin CS. Venous thromboembolism in cirrhosis: A review of the literature. Canadian Journal of Gastroenterology. 2012;**26**: 905-908

[121] Potze W, Arshad F, Adelmeijer J, Blokzijl H, van den Berg AP, Porte RJ, et al. Routine coagulation assays underestimate levels of antithrombin-dependent drugs but not of direct anticoagulant drugs in plasma from patients with cirrhosis. British Journal of Haematology. 2013;**163**:666-673

[122] Meduri GU, Kohler G, Headley S, Tolley E, Stentz F, Postlethwaite A. Inflammatory cytokines in the BAL of patients with ARDS: Persistent elevation over time predicts poor outcome. Chest. 1995;**108**:1303-1314

[123] Henderson LA, Canna SW, Schulert GS, Volpi S, Lee PY, Kernan KF, et al. On the alert for cytokine storm: Immunopathology in COVID-19. Arthritis Rheumatol. 2020 Jul;**72**(7): 1059-1063.

[124] José RJ, Williams AE, Chambers RC. Proteinase-activated receptors in fibroproliferative lung disease. Thorax. 2014;**69**:190-192

[125] Qamar A, Vaduganathan M, Greenberger NJ, Giugliano RP. Oral anticoagulation in patients with liver disease. Journal of the American College of Cardiology. 2018;**71**:2162-2175

[126] Hum J, Shatzel JJ, Jou JH, Deloughery TG. The efficacy and safety of direct oral anticoagulants vs traditional anticoagulants in cirrhosis. European Journal of Haematology. 2017;**98**:393-397

[127] Kuderer NM, Ortel TL, Francis CW. Impact of venous thromboembolism and anticoagulation on cancer and cancer survival. Journal of Clinical Oncology. 2009;**27**:4902

[128] Khorana A, Francis C, Culakova E, Kuderer N, Lyman G. Thromboembolism is a leading cause of death in cancer patients receiving outpatient chemotherapy. Journal of Thrombosis and Haemostasis. 2007;**5**:632-634

[129] Lyman GH, Bohlke K, Khorana AA, Kuderer NM, Lee AY, Arcelus JI, et al. Venous thromboembolism prophylaxis and treatment in patients with cancer: American Society of Clinical Oncology clinical practice guideline update 2014. Journal of Clinical Oncology. 2015; **33**:654

[130] Lee AY, Kamphuisen PW, Meyer G, Bauersachs R, Janas MS, Jarner MF, et al. Tinzaparin vs warfarin for treatment of acute venous thromboembolism in patients with active cancer: A randomized clinical trial. JAMA. 2015;**314**:677-686

[131] Lee AY, Levine MN, Baker RI, Bowden C, Kakkar AK, Prins M, et al. Low-molecular-weight heparin versus a coumarin for the prevention of recurrent venous thromboembolism in patients with cancer. The New England Journal of Medicine. 2003;**349**:146-153

[132] Bikdeli B, Madhavan MV, Jimenez D, Chuich T, Dreyfus I, Driggin E, et al. COVID-19 and thrombotic or thromboembolic disease: Implications for prevention, antithrombotic therapy, and follow-up: JACC state-of-the-art review. Journal of the American College of Cardiology. 2020;**75**:2950-2973

Chapter 5

Thrombolytic Therapy in Pulmonary Thromboembolism

Navdeep Singh Sidhu and Sumandeep Kaur

Abstract

Acute pulmonary thromboembolism (PE) is a common disorder with significant mortality and morbidity. Timely recognition and prompt therapy of this disorder is essential to prevent adverse consequences. Thrombolytic therapy has an important role in the management of high-risk pulmonary embolism patients, where it can be lifesaving. However, the potential clinical benefit of thrombolytic therapy needs to balanced against the risk of major bleeding associated with the use of these agents. Hence patient selection is of paramount importance in determining the success of this therapy. Management strategies in PE are centered around the concept of risk stratification of the cases. In this chapter we briefly discuss the risk categorization of PE cases, followed by a more elaborative discussion of the role of thrombolytic therapy in the management of patients with high risk or intermediate risk PE.

Keywords: pulmonary thromboembolism, embolism, thrombolysis, massive, high risk, sub-massive, intermediate risk, low risk, reperfusion, coronavirus, Covid-19

1. Introduction

Acute pulmonary thromboembolism (PE) is a frequent, often under-diagnosed disease with substantial in-hospital mortality and significant acute as well as long-term morbidity. Worldwide, venous thromboembolism (VTE), comprising of deep vein thrombosis (DVT) and PE, is the third most common acute cardiovascular syndrome after myocardial infarction and stroke [1]. The annual incidence rates of PE vary from 39 to 115 per 100,000 population and of DVT vary from 53 to 162 per 100,000 population, as estimated in epidemiological studies [2, 3]. Following the introduction of widespread use of D-dimer testing and computed tomography pulmonary angiography (CTPA) in 1990s, the estimated incidence of PE has increased significantly. A nationwide time trend analysis from United States has shown a substantial increase in incidence of PE after introduction of CTPA (81% increase, from 62.1 to 112.3 per 100,000) [4]. Other longitudinal studies have shown a similar trend with increased rates of PE over time [5]. The overall incidence rates of PE are higher in males as compared to females (56 versus 48 per 100,000, respectively) [6, 7]. The incidence rates increase exponentially with increasing age, especially in women, such that rates are nearly eight times higher in individuals aged >80 years than in the fifth decade of life [2].

Pulmonary embolism ranks third among the causes of cardiovascular death, after myocardial infarction and stroke [3]. It is one of the leading preventable causes of death in hospitalized patients. In the United States, PE is responsible for nearly 100,000 deaths annually [3, 6–9]. Data from six European countries with a total population of 454.4 million, has shown that in 2004, more than 370,000 deaths were related to VTE [8]. Of these, 34% died abruptly, or within the first few hours of an acute event, before treatment could be started or take effect. In other patients, mortality resulted from acute PE that was diagnosed after death in 59% and in only 7% of the patients who died early, the correct diagnosis of PE was made before death [8]. Time trend analyses from North American, European, and Asian populations have suggested that case fatality rates of acute PE may be declining [3, 10–15]. This positive impact on prognosis of acute PE appears to be related to more widespread use of effective therapies and interventions in the recent years [16, 17].

Prognosis from acute PE is related to the degree of obstruction and its hemodynamic consequences. According to its severity, PE is usually divided into 3 categories as proposed by American Heart Association (AHA) and European Society of Cardiology (ESC) guidelines [18, 19]:

1. Massive (AHA) or high risk (ESC) PE: these hemodynamically unstable patients are characterized by the presence of cardiac arrest or persistent hypotension [defined as a systolic blood pressure (SBP) <90 mmHg and/or a fall in SBP of >40 mmHg for at least 15 minutes, or needing vasopressor support], with or without the evidence of end organ hypo-perfusion. These patients account for nearly 5% of hospitalized PE patients and have an average one-month mortality of around 30% [20].

2. Sub-massive (AHA) or intermediate risk (ESC) PE: These patients are identified by the presence of right ventricle (RV) strain without hypotension. RV strain includes RV dysfunction on echocardiography or CTPA [right/left ventricular (LV) ratio > 0.9] or RV injury and pressure overload with an increase in the level of cardiac biomarkers like troponins or brain natriuretic peptide (BNP). There are some differences in the AHA and ESC guidelines pertaining to this category of patients. The criterion for sub-massive PE in AHA guidelines is the presence of RV strain without hypotension. The ESC criteria of intermediate-risk PE are more broader and include patients with a simplified Pulmonary Embolism Severity Index (sPESI) score ≥ 1 (i.e., age > 80 years; cancer, chronic heart failure or chronic pulmonary disease; heart rate > 110 bpm; SBP <100 mm Hg; or arterial oxygen saturation < 90%), regardless of presence of RV strain. The ESC further subcategorizes these patients into 2 sub-groups depending on the presence of both RV dysfunction and RV injury (intermediate risk—high) or only one or neither of these (intermediate risk—low). These patients with sub-massive or intermediate-risk PE constitute about 35–55% of hospitalized PE patients and the short-term mortality rates in this heterogeneous group vary from 2 to 3% over a period of 7 to 30 days in prospective randomized clinical trials [21], to 3–15% over a period of 7 to 90 days in observational cohort studies [22–24].

3. Low risk (AHA and ESC) PE: These are the patients of PE who do not meet the criteria for sub-massive (AHA) or intermediate-risk (ESC) PE. These account for 40–60% of hospitalized PE patients and have an estimated mortality of around 1% within 1 month [25].

Timely risk stratification of a patient with acute PE is essential for determining the optimal therapeutic approach. Low risk PE patients are typically managed with anticoagulation alone. In massive or high-risk PE patients and some selected high-risk patients in the sub-massive or intermediate risk category early reperfusion therapy is the need of hour, which can be lifesaving. Primary reperfusion therapy in most cases is systemic thrombolysis. Alternative reperfusion therapies include surgical embolectomy or percutaneous catheter-directed treatments, which are primarily used in patients with contraindications to systemic thrombolysis, depending upon the local availability and expertise [19]. In the following sections, we discuss the role of systemic thrombosis in the treatment of acute PE.

2. Use of thrombolytic therapy in acute pulmonary embolism

2.1 Decision to thrombolyse

In pulmonary embolism, thromboembolic obstruction of the pulmonary arterial tree with the resultant increase in right ventricular afterload is the central pathophysiologic process leading to the development of hemodynamic instability and possible mortality. Rapid removal of the clot, either pharmacologically or surgically results in prompt restoration of pulmonary circulation and decrease in pulmonary arterial pressures [26]. Thrombolysis has been shown to result in more rapid restoration of pulmonary perfusion as compared to anticoagulation alone, with resultant improvement in hemodynamics and right ventricular function. This positive impact of thrombosis on hemodynamics is limited to the initial few days. In patients surviving acute PE, these differences are no longer noted at one week after the therapy [27].

Decision to thrombolyse a patient with acute PE is of critical importance which requires a good judgment about the benefit–risk ratio of thrombolytic therapy. Instituting thrombolytic therapy in a sick patient with persistent hypotension or shock who is at low bleeding risk can prevent a potential mortality; whereas its use in an intermediate risk patient with high bleeding risk can have devastating bleeding consequences. Given the inherent difficulties in this decision making, many centers and society guidelines have advocated the formation of Pulmonary Embolism Response Teams (PERTs) for the management of high risk and selected cases of intermediate risk PE patients [19]. These teams could consist of specialists from different fields like cardiology, pulmonary, intensive care/anesthesiology, hematology, cardiac surgery, vascular medicine and interventional radiology, depending upon the local availability. This facilitates timely decision making in a particular case, with quick formulation of a treatment strategy and its implementation.

Thrombolysis is typically considered in a hemodynamically unstable patient who has a confirmed or highly suspected acute PE and who has a favorable risk–benefit ratio with a low bleeding risk. Diagnosis is usually made on the basis of findings of CTPA, although, ventilation-perfusion scans or catheter pulmonary angiography can also be confirmatory. Sometimes, the thrombolytic therapy is instituted on making the diagnosis by a bedside echocardiogram when patient is too sick to be shifted for CTPA or if it is not available immediately. Very infrequently, thrombolytic therapy may be started during cardiopulmonary resuscitation in a patient with high clinical suspicion of PE, although it is rarely effective in cases of refractory pulseless activity arrest.

Thrombolysis in PE is most effective when stated within 48 hours of symptom onset, but can still be potentially useful for up to 14 days of symptom onset in selected patients [19].

2.2 Thrombolysis in massive or high-risk PE

The most widely accepted indication of thrombolysis in acute PE is the presence of high risk or massive PE [18, 19, 28, 29]. These recommendations are supported by the findings of a small randomized controlled trial which compared thrombolytic therapy (streptokinase) followed by heparin or heparin alone in eight patients with massive PE. In this study, the thrombolytic therapy was found to be associated with significant reduction in mortality as compared to heparin alone [30].

2.3 Thrombolysis in sub-massive or intermediate risk PE

Thrombolysis in this category of PE is controversial and often requires an individualized approach to the patient. The current evidence does not support the routine use of thrombolytic therapy in these patients, although rescue thrombolysis is indicated in patients who have hemodynamic deterioration while being treated with anticoagulants [18, 19, 28, 29].

Nevertheless, thrombolysis in these patients has been associated with reduced chances of hemodynamic compromise and possibly, reduced risk of long-term complications including chronic thromboembolic pulmonary hypertension (CTEPH) [31], albeit, at the cost of increased bleeding events including intracranial hemorrhage.

There have been many studies which have tried to explore the role of thrombolytic therapy in this group of patients. The largest among these is the Pulmonary Embolism Thrombolysis (PEITHO) trial, a randomized double blind trial of 1005 patients [31]. It randomized normotensive patients with intermediate risk PE to either tenecteplase plus heparin or placebo plus heparin. To be eligible for this trial, the intermediate risk PE patients needed to have evidence of right ventricular dysfunction on echocardiography or CTPA along with elevated levels of cardiac troponins. The primary outcome of death or the development of hemodynamic compromise within 7 days occurred in 2.6% of the patients in tenecteplase group as compared to 5.6% in the placebo group (odds ratio, 0.44; 95% confidence interval, 0.23 to 0.87; p = 0.02). Up to 7 days of randomization, the mortality was not significant different between the groups (1.2% in tenecteplase group vs. 1.8% in placebo group, p = 0.42). The benefit of decreased primary outcome in this study came at the cost increased risk of major extra-cranial (6.2% in tenecteplase group vs. 1.2% in placebo group, p < 0.001) and intra-cranial bleeding (2% in tenecteplase group vs. 0.2% in placebo group, p = .003). On follow-up of up to 30 days, the death rate was not statistically significant between the groups (2.4% in tenecteplase group vs. 3.2% in placebo group, p = 0.42). Thus, in this study thrombolytic therapy decreased the incidence of development of hemodynamic compromise but had no impact on 7 days and 30 days mortality.

Other studies conducted in this field have been limited by smaller sample size of the study population, thus necessitating the use of composite outcome end-points. The management strategies and prognosis of pulmonary embolism (MAPPET-3) trial randomized 256 normotensive PE patients with pulmonary hypertension or RV dysfunction to receive either heparin plus alteplase or heparin plus placebo. The primary outcome of in-hospital mortality or clinical deterioration requiring an escalation of treatment, was significantly lower in thrombolytic group (11% vs. 24.6%, p = 0.006), and the thrombolytic group had higher the probability of 30-day event free survival by Kaplan-Meir estimates (p = 0.005). The difference in the primary outcome was largely due to higher number of patients in the heparin group requiring escalation of the treatment, with no significant difference in mortality. The incidence of fatal bleeding or hemorrhagic stroke was not significantly different between the groups [32]. Moderate Pulmonary Embolism Treated with Thrombolysis (MOPETT Trial) randomized 121 patients with moderate PE to receive low dose thrombolytic therapy plus anticoagulation or anticoagulation alone. In this study, the thrombolytic therapy was associated with a significant reduction of pulmonary hypertension which was maintained up to

28 months, although there was no difference in mortality [33]. The North American Tenecteplase or Placebo: Cardiopulmonary Outcomes at Three Months (TOPCOAT) trial also explored the use of thrombolytic therapy in patients with sub-massive PE [34]. This study had different design as compared to the contemporary PEITHO trial with broader definition of submissive PE which allowed inclusion if there was evidence of RV hypokinesis on echocardiography or there were elevated cardiac biomarkers (cardiac troponin I/T or BNP/NT-pro BNP). This trial had to be prematurely terminated due to relocation of the principal investigator and thus only 83 patients could be randomized. The primary outcome at 5 days (a composite of death, circulatory shock, intubation, or major bleeding) was seen in one patient in thrombolytic arm and three patients in the heparin arm.

There have been many systematic reviews and meta-analyses published regarding the use of thrombolysis in patients with sub-massive or intermediate PE. One such analysis by Chatterjee et al. in 2014, included 16 RCTs with 2115 patients of both massive (or high risk) and sub-massive (or intermediate risk) PE patients. This analysis reported a lower all-cause mortality in thrombolytic group (odds ratio 0.53, 95% confidence intervals 0.32–0.88), although with a greater risk of major bleeding (odds ratio 2.73, 95% confidence intervals 1.91–3.91). In a sub-set of 1775 patients from 8 trials of intermediate risk PE, it was noted that systemic thrombolytic therapy was associated with reduction in mortality in intermediate high-risk PE patients with RV dysfunction as compared to anticoagulation alone (odds ratio 0.48, 95% confidence intervals 0.25–0.92), but at the cost of increased major bleeding events (odds ratio 3.19, 95% confidence intervals 2.07–4.92) [21]. A recently published meta-analysis by Zuo et al. in 2021, included 21 trials with a total of 2401 patients with both stable and unstable PE. The results showed that thrombolytic therapy followed by heparin was associated with lower risk of death (odds ratio 0.58, 95% confidence intervals 0.38–0.88) and recurrent PE (odds ratio 0.54, 95% confidence interval 0.32–0.91). However, the evidence was of low certainty for both of these outcomes as the effects weakened significantly after the exclusion of one study with high risk of bias. Thrombolytic therapy was associated with higher risk of major bleeding (odds ratio 2.84, 95% confidence intervals 1.92–4.20) and hemorrhagic stroke (odds ratio 7.59, 95% confidence intervals 1.38–41.72) [35].

Given the equivocal nature of the clinical evidence till date, the decision to thrombolyse a patient with sub-massive or intermediate PE should be individualized with careful consideration of the benefit–risk ratio. The AHA 2011 guidelines support the use of thrombolytic therapy in sub-massive PE cases who have clinical evidence of adverse prognosis (new hemodynamic instability, deteriorating respiratory failure, severe RV dysfunction, or major myocardial necrosis) and low risk of bleeding (Class IIb; Level of Evidence C) [18]. The 2016 CHEST guidelines recommend against the use of thrombolytic therapy in acute PE without hypotension (grade 1B) [28]. Similarly, the ESC 2019 guidelines and 2020 American Society of Hematology (ASH) guidelines recommend against the routine use of thrombolytic therapy in patients with intermediate risk or sub-massive PE [19, 29].

2.4 Thrombolytic agents and their dosing

The approved thrombolytic agents and their dosing in PE has been shown in **Table 1**.

To date, no studies have been shown the superiority of one agent over the other in this patient population. The ease of administration coupled with the non-availability of first-generation agents (streptokinase and urokinase), has made recombinant tissue-plasminogen activator (rt-PA, alteplase) as the favored agents in most of the developed world; however, given their lower costs, the first-generation agents are still

Drug	Dose
Recombinant tissue-plasminogen activator (rt-PA)	100 mg in 2 hours, accelerated regimen 0.6 mg/kg over 15 mins (maximum dose 50 mg)
Streptokinase	250,000 IU loading dose over 30 mins, followed by 100,000 IU/h for 12–24 h; accelerated regimen 1.5 million IU over 2 h
Urokinase	4400 IU loading dose over 10 mins, followed by 4400 IU/kg/h over 12–24 h; accelerated regimen: 3 million IU over 2 h

Table 1.
Approved thrombolytic agents and their dosing in pulmonary embolism [19].

widely used in the developing world. Unfractionated heparin (UFH) may be continued during the infusion of rt-PA but it should be with-held during the infusion of strep-tokinase or urokinase [19]. Other investigational thrombolytic agents for use in PE include tenecteplase, reteplase, desmoteplase, but none has been approved as yet [19].

2.5 Contraindications to thrombolysis

The major contraindications to thrombolytic therapy are listed in **Table 2**.

Absolute contraindications
• History of hemorrhagic stroke or stroke of unknown origin
• Ischemic stroke in last 6 months
• Intracranial neoplasm or structural cerebral vascular lesion
• Major trauma, surgery or head injury in last 3 weeks
• Active bleeding (excluding menstrual bleeding)
• Bleeding diathesis
• Suspected aortic dissection
Relative contraindications
• Severe uncontrolled hypertension (systolic BP >180 mm Hg or diastolic BP >110 mm Hg)
• History of poor controlled hypertension in the past
• Transient ischemic attack in last 6 months
• Current use of oral anticoagulants
• Pregnancy or first week post-partum
• Non-compressible vascular puncture sites
• Age more than 75 years
• Advanced liver disease
• Active peptic ulcer disease
• For streptokinase or urokinase: previous exposure (more than 5 days ago) or previous allergic reaction to these agents

Table 2.
Contraindications to thrombolysis [18, 19].

2.6 Assessment of response to therapy

This is usually done by continued clinical monitoring of the patient for improvement in signs and symptoms (e.g., improved blood pressure, reduced respiratory rate or heart rate, improvement in oxygenation). Some centers advocate serial echocardiograms to evaluate for improvements in pulmonary artery pressures and RV dysfunction. Although RV size and function may improve acutely, but often it may lag behind the signs of clinical improvement by several weeks to months. After thrombolytic therapy the patient is transitioned to long term anticoagulant therapy depending upon the etiology.

2.7 Role of low dose thrombolytic therapy

The disappointingly high rates of intra-cranial hemorrhage in the PEITHO trial, led many investigators to explore the use of low-dose thrombolytic therapy in patients with PE. The widely recommended rt-PA dose of 100 mg over 2 hours is largely based from experience from the patients with myocardial infarction. Many researchers have argued that lungs may be an organ with higher sensitivity to thrombolytic therapy as compared to the myocardium and given that lungs receive the entirety of cardiac output as compared to only 5% being received by the coronary circulation, low-dose thrombolytic therapy in PE seems to be a logical approach. Low-doses thrombolytic therapy could be especially useful in elderly patients, pregnant patients and in those who have relative contraindications.

A multicenter RCT by China VTE group published in 2010, randomized 118 patients with either hemodynamic unstable or anatomic massive pulmonary obstruction to full dose (100 mg/2 h) rt-PA regimen or half dose (50 mg/h) rt-PA regimen. Half-dose regimen was associated with similar improvements in RV function, lung perfusion defects and pulmonary artery obstruction, and had lesser bleeding complications especially in patients with body weight of less than 65 kgs [36]. The subsequent MOPETT trial (as described above) published in 2013, demonstrated significant lower risk of progressive pulmonary hypertension in low-dose thrombolytic arm, albeit with a similar mortality [34]. Another study of 66 patients with intermediate risk PE, randomized patients to receive either low dose rt-PA (30 mg/2 h) plus low-molecular weight heparin (LMWH) or LMWH alone. In this study, the thrombolytic group had significant reductions in pulmonary artery systolic pressures (PASP) and the RV/LV ratio as compared to the baseline. There was no significant change in these parameters from the baseline in LMWH group. Thrombolytic therapy resulted in significant decrease in PASP and an improved symptom severity as compared to LMWH group. On follow up of 90 days, no significant difference was noted in terms of mortality, recurrent venous thromboembolism or major bleeding, although, thrombolytic group had more minor bleeding and less hemodynamic decompensation [37]. In a recently published prospective, non-randomized open label, single center study of 76 patients with intermediate risk PE, half dose rt-PA (50 mg/2 h) plus LMWH was compared to LMWH alone. It was found that half dose rt-PA significantly prevented mortality or hemodynamic deterioration at 7 days and 30 days without increase in bleeding risk [38]. Thus, the results from these small studies suggest that low dose thrombolytic therapy may be an attractive option in the treatment of PE, however, larger RCTs are needed to draw definite conclusions on this topic.

2.8 Thrombolysis in pulmonary embolism related to Covid-19

Coronavirus disease-19 (Covid-19) is associated with a significantly increased risk of procoagulant events including PE, the risk being highest in critically ill patients with severe disease admitted to intensive care units (ICUs) [39]. The development of PE in patients with Covid-19 is associated with worse outcomes, mandating quick recognition and prompt management [40]. In the absence of robust data from large studies, the Global COVID-19 Thrombosis Collaborative Group currently advocates managing PE in Covid-19 on the similar lines as patients of non-Covid PE [41]. Systemic thrombolysis is recommended for patients with Covid-19 related PE in case of massive or high-risk PE; or in patients with sub-massive or intermediate PE who develop hemodynamic deterioration while being treated with anticoagulant therapy. However, there are few peculiarities of this situation which demand careful consideration. Firstly, it is often difficult to disentangle the hemodynamic consequences of PE in a sick Covid-19 patient from those of severe pneumonia and acute respiratory distress syndrome (ARDS); thus, necessitating critical thinking and judgment. Secondly, Covid-19 is often associated with an unfamiliar coagulopathy with the presence of thrombocytopenia in a sizeable proportion of the patients which increases the risk of bleeding complications from systemic thrombolysis [42]. Presence of co-existent thrombocytopenia calls for an individualized approach in such patients and many researchers have advocated the use of catheter directed thrombolysis as the potential first line therapy in these patients [43]. Further evidence from larger studies is needed in this field to guide decision making.

3. Conclusions

Acute PE is a frequent disorder which needs timely recognition and management to ensure good outcomes. Thrombolytic therapy plays a central role in the management of patients with massive (or high-risk) PE, where it can be lifesaving. This therapy can also be useful in improving outcomes in carefully selected patients with sub-massive (or intermediate risk) PE.

Author details

Navdeep Singh Sidhu[1]* and Sumandeep Kaur[2]

1 Department of Cardiology, GGS Medical College and Baba Farid University of Health Sciences, Faridkot, Punjab, India

2 Faculty of Nursing Sciences, Baba Farid University of Health Sciences, Faridkot, Punjab, India

*Address all correspondence to: navsids@gmail.com

IntechOpen

References

[1] Raskob GE, Angchaisuksiri P, Blanco AN, Buller H, Gallus A, Hunt BJ, et al. Thrombosis: a major contributor to global disease burden. Arteriosclerosis, Thrombosis, and Vascular Biology. 2014;**34**:23632371

[2] Wendelboe AM, Raskob GE. Global burden of thrombosis: epidemiologic aspects. Circulation Research. 2016;**118**:13401347

[3] Keller K, Hobohm L, Ebner M, Kresoja KP, Munzel T, Konstantinides SV, et al. Trends in thrombolytic treatment and outcomes of acute pulmonary embolism in Germany. European Heart Journal. 2020;**41**:522529

[4] Wiener RS, Schwartz LM, Woloshin S. Time trends in pulmonary embolism in the United States: evidence of overdiagnosis. Archives of Internal Medicine. 2011;**171**:831

[5] Konstantinides SV. Trends in incidence versus case fatality rates of pulmonary embolism: Good news or bad news? Thrombosis and Haemostasis. 2016;**115**:233

[6] Horlander KT, Mannino DM, Leeper KV. Pulmonary embolism mortality in the United States, 1979-1998: an analysis using multiple-cause mortality data. Archives of Internal Medicine. 2003;**163**:1711

[7] Naess IA, Christiansen SC, Romundstad P, Cannegieter SC, Rosendaal FR, Hammerstrøm J. Incidence and mortality of venous thrombosis: a population-based study. Journal of Thrombosis and Haemostasis. 2007 Apr;**5**(4):692-699. DOI: 10.1111/j.1538-7836.2007.02450.x

[8] Tagalakis V, Patenaude V, Kahn SR, Suissa S. Incidence of and mortality from venous thromboembolism in a real-world population: the Q-VTE Study Cohort. Am J Med 2013; 126:832.e13

[9] Lassila R, Jula A, Pitkäniemi J, Haukka J. The association of statin use with reduced incidence of venous thromboembolism: a population-based cohort study. BMJ Open 2014; 4:e005862

[10] Cohen AT, Agnelli G, Anderson FA, Arcelus JI, Bergqvist D, Brecht JG, et al; VTE Impact Assessment Group in Europe (VITAE). Venous thromboembolism (VTE) in Europe. The number of VTE events and associated morbidity and mortality. Thrombosis and Haemostasis 2007;**98**:756764

[11] de Miguel-Diez J, Jimenez-Garcia R, Jimenez D, Monreal M, Guijarro R, Otero R, et al. Trends in hospital admissions for pulmonary embolism in Spain from 2002 to 2011. The European Respiratory Journal. 2014;**44**:942950

[12] Dentali F, Ageno W, Pomero F, Fenoglio L, Squizzato A, Bonzini M. Time trends and case fatality rate of in-hospital treated pulmonary embolism during 11 years of observation in Northwestern Italy. Thrombosis and Haemostasis. 2016;**115**:399405

[13] Lehnert P, Lange T, Moller CH, Olsen PS, Carlsen J. Acute pulmonary embolism in a national Danish cohort: increasing incidence and decreasing mortality. Thrombosis and Haemostasis. 2018;**118**:539546

[14] Jimenez D, de Miguel-Diez J, Guijarro R, Trujillo-Santos J, Otero R. Barba R, et al. RIETE Investigators. Trends in the management and outcomes of acute pulmonary embolism: analysis from the RIETE registry. J Am Coll Cardiol. 2016;**67**: 162170

[15] Agarwal S, Clark D III, Sud K, Jaber WA, Cho L, Menon V. Gender disparities in outcomes and resource utilization for acute pulmonary embolism hospitalizations in the United States. The American Journal of Cardiology. 2015;**116**:12701276

[16] Roy PM, Meyer G, Vielle B, Le Gall C, Verschuren F. Carpentier F, et al. EMDEPU Study Group. Appropriateness of diagnostic management and outcomes of suspected pulmonary embolism. Ann Intern Med. 2006;**144**:157164

[17] Jimenez D, Bikdeli B, Barrios D, Morillo R, Nieto R. Guerassimova I, et al. RIETE Investigators. Management appropriateness and outcomes of patients with acute pulmonary embolism. Eur Respir J. 2018;**51**:1800445

[18] Jaff MR, McMurtry MS, Archer SL, Cushman M, Goldenberg N, Goldhaber SZ, et al; on behalf of the American Heart Association Council on Cardiopulmonary, Critical Care, Perioperative and Resuscitation; American Heart Association Council on Peripheral Vascular Disease; American Heart Association Council on Arteriosclerosis, Thrombosis and Vascular Biology. Management of massive and submassive pulmonary embolism, iliofemoral deep vein thrombosis, and chronic thromboembolic pulmonary hypertension: a scientific statement from the American Heart Association [published corrections appear in Circulation. 2012;125:e496 and Circulation. 2012;126:e495]. Circulation. 2011;123:1788-1830. doi: 10.1161/CIR.0b013e318214914f

[19] Konstantinides SV, Meyer G, Becattini C, Bueno H, Geersing GJ, Harjola VP. et al; ESC Scientific Document Group. 2019 ESC Guidelines for the diagnosis and management of acute pulmonary embolism developed in collaboration with the European Respiratory Society (ERS). European Heart Journal. 2020 Jan 21;**41**(4): 543-603. DOI: 10.1093/eurheartj/ehz405

[20] Vanni S, Nazerian P, Pepe G, Baioni M, Risso M, Grifoni G, et al. Comparison of two prognostic models for acute pulmonary embolism: clinical vs. right ventricular dysfunction-guided approach. Journal of Thrombosis and Haemostasis. 2011;**9**:1916-1923. DOI: 10.1111/j.1538-7836.2011.04459.x

[21] Chatterjee S, Chakraborty A, Weinberg I, Kadakia M, Wilensky RL, Sardar P, et al. Thrombolysis for pulmonary embolism and risk of all-cause mortality, major bleeding, and intracranial hemorrhage: a meta-analysis. Journal of the American Medical Association. 2014;**311**:2414-2421. DOI: 10.1001/jama.2014.5990

[22] Becattini C, Agnelli G. Predictors of mortality from pulmonary embolism and their influence on clinical management. Thromb Haemost. 2008;100:747-751. 20

[23] Lin BW, Schreiber DH, Liu G, Briese B, Hiestand B, Slattery D, et al. Therapy and outcomes in massive pulmonary embolism from the Emergency Medicine Pulmonary Embolism in the Real World Registry. The American Journal of Emergency Medicine. 2012;**30**:1774-1781. DOI: 10.1016/j.ajem.2012.02.012

[24] Secemsky E, Chang Y, Jain CC, Beckman JA, Giri J, Jaff MR, et al. Contemporary management and outcomes of patients with massive and submassive pulmonary embolism. Am J Med. 2018;131:1506-1514.e0. doi: 10.1016/j.amjmed.2018.07.035

[25] Jiménez D, Kopecna D, Tapson V, Briese B, Schreiber D, Lobo JL. et al; PROTECT Investigators. Derivation and validation of multimarker prognostication for normotensive patients with acute symptomatic

pulmonary embolism. American Journal of Respiratory and Critical Care Medicine. 2014;**189**:718-726. DOI: 10.1164/rccm.201311-2040OC

[26] Becattini C, Agnelli G, Salvi A, Grifoni S, Pancaldi LG, Enea I, et al. Bolus tenecteplase for right ventricle dysfunction in hemodynamically stable patients with pulmonary embolism. Thrombosis Research. 2010 Mar;**125**(3):e82-e86. DOI: 10.1016/j.thromres.2009.09.017

[27] Dalla-Volta S, Palla A, Santolicandro A, Giuntini C, Pengo V, Visioli O, et al. PAIMS 2: alteplase combined with heparin versus heparin in the treatment of acute pulmonary embolism. Plasminogen activator Italian multicenter study 2. Journal of the American College of Cardiology. 1992 Sep;**20**(3):520-526. DOI: 10.1016/0735-1097(92)90002-5

[28] Kearon C, Akl EA, Ornelas J, Blaivas A, Jimenez D, Bounameaux H, et al. Antithrombotic Therapy for VTE Disease: CHEST Guideline and Expert Panel Report. Chest. 2016 Feb;**149**(2):315-352. DOI: 10.1016/j.chest.2015.11.026

[29] Ortel TL, Neumann I, Ageno W, Beyth R, Clark NP, Cuker A, et al. American Society of Hematology 2020 guidelines for management of venous thromboembolism: treatment of deep vein thrombosis and pulmonary embolism. Blood Advances. 2020 Oct 13;**4**(19):4693-4738. DOI: 10.1182/bloodadvances.2020001830

[30] Jerjes-Sanchez C, Ramírez-Rivera A, de Lourdes GM, Arriaga-Nava R, Valencia S, Rosado-Buzzo A, et al. Streptokinase and Heparin versus Heparin Alone in Massive Pulmonary Embolism: A Randomized Controlled Trial. Journal of Thrombosis and Thrombolysis. 1995;**2**(3):227-229. DOI: 10.1007/BF01062714

[31] Meyer G, Vicaut E, Danays T, Agnelli G, Becattini C, Beyer-Westendorf J. et al; PEITHO Investigators. Fibrinolysis for patients with intermediate-risk pulmonary embolism. The New England Journal of Medicine. 2014 Apr 10;**370**(15):1402-1411. DOI: 10.1056/NEJMoa1302097

[32] Konstantinides S, Geibel A, Heusel G, Heinrich F. Kasper W; Management Strategies and Prognosis of Pulmonary Embolism-3 Trial Investigators. Heparin plus alteplase compared with heparin alone in patients with submassive pulmonary embolism. The New England Journal of Medicine. 2002 Oct 10;**347**(15):1143-1150. DOI: 10.1056/NEJMoa021274

[33] Sharifi M, Bay C, Skrocki L, Rahimi F. Mehdipour M; "MOPETT" Investigators. Moderate pulmonary embolism treated with thrombolysis (from the "MOPETT" Trial). The American Journal of Cardiology. 2013 Jan 15;**111**(2):273-277. DOI: 10.1016/j.amjcard.2012.09.027

[34] Kline JA, Nordenholz KE, Courtney DM, Kabrhel C, Jones AE, Rondina MT, et al. Treatment of submassive pulmonary embolism with tenecteplase or placebo: cardiopulmonary outcomes at 3 months: multicenter double-blind, placebo-controlled randomized trial. Journal of Thrombosis and Haemostasis. 2014 Apr;**12**(4):459-468. DOI: 10.1111/jth.12521

[35] Zuo Z, Yue J, Dong BR, Wu T, Liu GJ, Hao Q. Thrombolytic therapy for pulmonary embolism. Cochrane Database of Systematic Reviews 2021 Apr 15;**4**(4):CD004437. doi: 10.1002/14651858.CD004437

[36] Wang C, Zhai Z, Yang Y, Wu Q, Cheng Z, Liang L. et al; China Venous Thromboembolism (VTE) Study Group. Efficacy and safety of low dose recombinant tissue-type plasminogen

activator for the treatment of acute pulmonary thromboembolism: a randomized, multicenter, controlled trial. Chest. 2010 Feb;**137**(2):254-262. DOI: 10.1378/chest.09-0765

[37] Zhang LY, Gao BA, Jin Z, Xiang GM, Gong Z, Zhang TT, et al. Clinical efficacy of low dose recombinant tissue-type plasminogen activator for the treatment of acute intermediate-risk pulmonary embolism. Saudi Med J. 2018 Nov;39(11):1090-1095. doi: 10.15537/smj.2018.11.22717

[38] Yilmaz ES, Uzun O. Low-dose thrombolysis for submassive pulmonary embolism. J Investig Med. 2021 Jun 7:jim-2021-001816. doi: 10.1136/jim-2021-001816

[39] Tan BK, Mainbourg S, Friggeri A, Bertoletti L, Douplat M, Dargaud Y, et al. Arterial and venous thromboembolism in COVID-19: a study-level meta-analysis. Thorax. 2021 Oct;**76**(10):970-979. DOI: 10.1136/thoraxjnl-2020-215383

[40] Sakr Y, Giovini M, Leone M, Pizzilli G, Kortgen A, Bauer M, et al. Pulmonary embolism in patients with coronavirus disease-2019 (COVID-19) pneumonia: a narrative review. Annals of Intensive Care. 2020 Sep 16;**10**:124. DOI: 10.1186/s13613-020-00741-0

[41] Bikdeli B, Madhavan MV, Jimenez D, Chuich T, Dreyfus I, Driggin E. et al; Global COVID-19 Thrombosis Collaborative Group, Endorsed by the ISTH, NATF, ESVM, and the IUA, Supported by the ESC Working Group on Pulmonary Circulation and Right Ventricular Function. COVID-19 and Thrombotic or Thromboembolic Disease: Implications for Prevention, Antithrombotic Therapy, and Follow-Up: JACC State-of-the-Art Review. Journal of the American College of Cardiology. 2020 Jun 16;**75**(23):2950-2973. DOI: 10.1016/j.jacc.2020.04.031

[42] Lippi G, Plebani M, Henry BM. Thrombocytopenia is associated with severe coronavirus disease 2019 (COVID-19) infections: a meta-analysis. Clinica Chimica Acta. 2020;**506**:145-148. DOI: 10.1016/j.cca.2020.03.022

[43] Roncon L, Zuin M, Zonzin P. Fibrinolysis in COVID-19 patients with hemodynamic unstable acute pulmonary embolism: yes or no? Journal of Thrombosis and Thrombolysis. 2020;**50**:221-222. DOI: 10.1007/s11239-020-02131-6

www.ingramcontent.com/pod-product-compliance
Lightning Source LLC
Chambersburg PA
CBHW081240190326
41458CB00016B/5860